'This is a tour de force and makes a huge co psychosynthesis. Aubyn unpacks the depth that want to work within a psychospiritual context t bring purpose and meaning to their lives and to ....p. His words are highly accessible as he helps us explore the alchemy of coaching the 'being' and suffering of soul as clients find themselves and free their will to enable change. A must-read for all coaches looking to make a real difference.'

Roger H. Evans, author of *The Creative Manager* and *5DL Five Dimensions of Leadership*, co-founder and Director of Coaching, the Institute of Psychosynthesis, London

'What a delight. We have long needed a book devoted to evolutionary psychosynthesis and holistic coaching. This rich book pays attention to what APECS calls CPPD, our personal and professional development, encouraging us to look at not only the complexities of the outer organisational world, but the complexities of our inner world such as our conflicting needs and motivations, creating synergy, and to put identity, purpose, meaning and values centre stage. Mixing psychosynthesis history with theory and practice, while also referring to other approaches, the reader benefits from both a grounding in the subject and ideas to implement. Howard successfully argues the need for a psycho-spiritual perspective for the "emerging and growing crisis of leadership" and takes us on a journey to integrate our whole selves to work with the whole self of the other. Working at the level of 'being' we increase our capacity and that of leaders to deal with complexity.'

Eve Turner, chair, APECS; co-founder, Climate Coaching Alliance; and founder/lead, Global Supervisors' Network

'Psychosynthesis leadership coaching has great value for the development of the young discipline of coaching, of which Roberto Assagioli, the founder of psychosynthesis, especially with his book *The Act of Will*, was an enlightened pioneer.

Aubyn Howard delivers to new and more experienced coaches, organisational leaders, human resources and organisational development professionals the precious legacy of psychosynthesis: an approach that has always been characterised by the tension to combine different active techniques and very solid methods of guidance to effective action with a deep, systemic and integrated vision of the human being that also takes into account our emotional and spiritual dimensions, higher values, creativity and free will. A vision which, as the author states, we are in great need in this "increasingly complex, uncertain and stressful world". Thank you Aubyn!'

Petra Guggisberg Nocelli, psychotherapist ASP, psychosynthesist SIPT, trainer and author of *The Way of Psychosynthesis*

'Aubyn Howard has masterfully blended the powerful models of psychosynthesis psychology with contemporary coaching practice in an accessible and readable way. This book will be of value equally to those working in organisational coaching and those working in the field of psychotherapy and personal growth.'

Keith Silvester, president of the European Federation for Psychosynthesis Psychotherapy

'In addition to making a worthy and much needed contribution to leadership, executive and organisational coaching, Aubyn clarifies where leadership coaching sits in the context of coaching, psychosynthesis and leadership. He acknowledges healthy diversity in the profession and clearly distinguishes it from therapy and life coaching. This seminal publication encourages joined-up thinking on relevant theory and practice. It is an essential read for those in or interested in the leadership coaching profession, for human resource managers and for leaders or those aspiring to become leaders.'

Ger Melia, diploma in 5DL coaching, MSc education management, executive coach, Ireland

'A lucid and enlivening introduction to psychosynthesis; its history, its nature and its potential. Howard illustrates theoretically and demonstrates practically how psychosynthesis offers a unique scale of development essential for today's leaders. This book is a gift to coaches and leaders alike.'

Ant Mitchell, founder of Mitchell Coaching; Director of APECS

'In this wise and comprehensive book Aubyn contextualises Psychosynthesis Leadership Coaching. It allows the reader to reflect deeply on their current practice and on their own psychospiritual development. In our landscape of complexity, crisis and conflict, this should be required reading for all coaches, leaders, human resource and leadership development professionals who want to work at the deepest levels with themselves and others to effect real and sustainable change.'

Nana-Efua Lawson, managing director and principal psychologist, Castlegate International and PGCPLC graduate

Psychosynthesis Leadership Coaching

Psychosynthesis Leadership Coaching responds to the call of coaches who want to be able to work with the whole person, with the inner as well as the outer worlds, and not just at rational and behavioural levels but at emotional and spiritual levels as well.

Psychosynthesis is unique amongst psychologies in the emphasis it places on *self* and *will* at the centre of human psychological functioning. This holistic and integrative psychology provides the foundations for working with leaders in ways that respond to today's emergent crises.

Psychosynthesis coaching is an increasingly popular approach that is finding its way into the mainstream as a response to the needs of coaching to engage at depth with emotional content and in the transpersonal realm of meaning, purpose and values. This book introduces psychosynthesis coaching to a wider audience and provides a comprehensive guide to this approach for both coaches and leaders.

This book provides the context, models, methods, skills and techniques for coaches to engage with their clients within the larger context of Self and Will, alongside working on inner and outer agendas and goals of any description. For coaches, leaders and organisational practitioners alike, this approach is also about coaching our inner leader – knowing that this work always starts with ourselves.

Aubyn Howard is the co-founder of Psychosynthesis Coaching Limited and holds an MA in Psychosynthesis Psychology and MSc in Change Agent Skills and Strategies. He draws upon more than 30 years' experience as an organisational consultant, facilitator and coach and is an APECS accredited executive coach. Aubyn lives in France with his wife Diana.

Psychosynthesis Leadership Coaching

A Psychology of Being for a Time of Crisis

Aubyn Howard

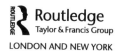

Routledge
Taylor & Francis Group

LONDON AND NEW YORK

First published 2021
by Routledge
2 Park Square, Milton Park, Abingdon, Oxon OX14 4RN

and by Routledge
52 Vanderbilt Avenue, New York, NY 10017

Routledge is an imprint of the Taylor & Francis Group, an informa business

British Library Cataloguing-in-Publication Data
A catalogue record for this book is available from the British Library

Library of Congress Cataloging-in-Publication Data
A catalog record has been requested for this book

ISBN: 978-1-138-54356-0 (hbk)
ISBN: 978-1-138-54357-7 (pbk)
ISBN: 978-1-351-00646-0 (ebk)

Typeset in Times New Roman
by Newgen Publishing UK

To the loving memory of both my mother, from whom I learned a love of learning, and my father, who gave me an inner critic who likes to make things clear.

Contents

Figures

Tables

Preface

Some background

I have written this book both because it was needed (and because I was invited to do so by Routledge) and also because I needed to write it as a way of externalising and synthesising my unfolding vision of psychosynthesis coaching.

Much of the material of the book has origins in my Master's thesis in psychosynthesis psychology completed in 2018, which, in turn, drew upon material from my online blog posts over the previous couple of years. However, the greatest inspiration has been the postgraduate certificate coaching courses that myself and Paul Elliott have run since 2015 and the profound personal and professional learning that I have experienced from working with our students on these.

Academically, the book provides an exposition of psychosynthesis coaching from three main perspectives: (i) from the point of view of coaching and why it benefits from being underpinned by such a psychology; (ii) from an understanding of the psychology of psychosynthesis and what it brings to coaching; and (iii) from the dynamic emergent needs of organisational leadership and what is being called for from coaches. The interplay of these perspectives creates the dynamic, emergent and developing model of psychosynthesis coaching that I will set out for the reader.

Coaching is a young and fast-developing field of professional practice within which there are many ideas and approaches competing for prominence and acceptance. Although psychosynthesis is an established and continuously evolving psychology in its own right, most of its application to professional practice has been in relationship to counselling and psychotherapy. We will describe the origins of psychosynthesis, including an overview of the life and work of Roberto Assagioli. We go on to trace developments in psychosynthesis coaching and how it is still embryonic and developing as a recognised approach or discipline. Historically, at least three different versions have emerged; (i) Roger Evans has been developing and practising his coaching approach for many decades, and the London Institute of Psychosynthesis has been training psychosynthesis coaches for more than a decade, culminating in the MA in psychosynthesis organisational and leadership coaching; (ii) Didi Firman and the Synthesis Center have been providing psychosynthesis life coach training for many years in the USA; and (iii) the late Sir John Whitmore referred increasingly explicitly to psychosynthesis coaching in each edition of his seminal book *Coaching for Performance* (see Part IV, 4th edition, 2009) and who included this perspective in both short courses and the Masters coaching programmes he was involved in.

Add to this mix the organisation that Paul Elliott and myself set up in 2015 to run shorter postgraduate certificate courses in partnership with the London Institute – Psychosynthesis Coaching Limited (PCL). In the creation and running of this programme, we have developed and enhanced the core model of psychosynthesis coaching and this process continues with each new programme.

Alongside this, the community of practising psychosynthesis coachees has been coming together, both formally and informally, in a process of reflective practitioner learning. PCL hosted the first Psychosynthesis Coaching Symposium in November 2018 in London, attended by sixty people from a variety of training backgrounds, and a second symposium in February 2020, this time attended by eighty people including a more international mix. There is a strong representation of psychosynthesis coaches within APECS, the top-level professional membership association for executive coaches, and psychosynthesis coaching features often and prominently at APECS learning events.

In addition, there is the unique story of how psychosynthesis coaching has been applied to internal coach development at GlaxoSmithKline, led in part by Anne Welsh and involving a cadre of other psychosynthesis coaches. It should also be said that probably most of the practising psychosynthesis coaches today didn't train specifically as psychosynthesis coaches, but trained in psychosynthesis (e.g. on the way to becoming a counsellor or therapist with the London Institute, the Psychosynthesis Trust or Re-Vision in the UK) and have combined this with other learning about coaching. Each of these coaches will have their own take on psychosynthesis coaching, depending upon the path they have followed.

Sir John Whitmore, in the fourth edition of his book *Coaching for Performance* (2009), dedicates the final part to transpersonal coaching and describes psychosynthesis coaching as a specialisation that enables coaches to work at greater depth and support leaders through the significant crises that can arise. However, until now, there has been no detailed or expansive text on this approach. This book picks up at the point at which John Whitmore leaves off and takes the coach into the territory of working not just at the transpersonal level, but at all levels of human consciousness.

One intention of this book is to create some coherence, alignment and clarity about psychosynthesis coaching without ignoring the diversity of experience or different perspectives that those involved in this field bring.

As much as possible within this, I try to acknowledge my own biases and preferences and point to other contributions where relevant. The version of psychosynthesis coaching that I will articulate here is offered not as the right version or the only version, but as one which I am co-creating with others and that is open to challenge or improvement. One important choice I am making at the outset is to focus on leadership, executive or organisational coaching rather than life coaching.

However, I will address the question about the distinction between life and leadership coaching, as well as the broader distinction between coaching and therapy, because these distinctions are important for the coaching practitioner in defining their field of competence and practice. In general, leadership coaching is a more complex domain of study than life coaching (e.g. involving the complexities of organisational systems, etc.), although there are aspects and dimensions to life coaching which are also challenging and would not be touched upon in a leadership coach training. Suffice to say, there are important questions about life coaching which I will not visit in this book, for example concerning the boundary between counselling and life coaching, and how counselling is giving ground to life coaching in the broader market for professional helping services.

This book is intended to fulfil different needs for different readers. For new or inexperienced coaches, it will open the doors to a whole new territory that is part of coaching, and provide some handrails for working at greater depth – as well as direction for their own personal and professional development. For more experienced and developed coaches, it may provide context, theory, models and ideas that can help them integrate and enhance their existing practice and learning. For organisational leaders, it may assist them to recognise critical issues and challenges at deeper levels, for both themselves and the people they lead, that are often not expressed or openly explored, and as a result help them find some ways to work with them. For human resources and organisational development professionals it could serve as an introduction to a psychospiritual psychology which has broader value in the development of leadership within their organisations.

Personal journey

My personal mission, simply stated, is to make psychosynthesis coaching more available and accessible to leaders within organisations and through these leaders to make a difference to organisational well-being, development and evolution. This mission underpinned my desire to establish Psychosynthesis Coaching Limited and the programmes we run in partnership with the Institute. This has been an unfolding and evolving passion over many years of involvement with psychosynthesis (since 2000). During my training at the London Institute, although I was applying psychosynthesis to my work as an organisational consultant, facilitator and coach, my primary focus was on my own healing process, which I characterised as resolving the split between my mind and my heart and becoming grounded in my being. Subsequently, during many years of working with Roger Evans in his consulting business with large organisational clients, my focus moved to the needs and issues of clients, to listening to the other and finding a way to authentically engage in the role of professional practitioner in complex organisational environments.

Since 2014, my focus has shifted to the wider challenge of bringing psycho-synthesis more fully into the organisational world and to the education and development of other leadership coaches. Through this recent period I have been able to reconnect with my will in a way that has led to a very rich period of continuing personal and professional development. In many significant ways this process of engaging in what has felt like my life's work has curiously and miraculously resolved unfinished business in the previous two periods – concerning my personal healing and my ability to work authentically with clients.

Alongside the themes I have already outlined above, there is a deeper thread running through this book concerning my own personal connection with Roberto Assagioli and his work, involving mystical and transpersonal currents beyond explicit narrative and immediate awareness. In researching and writing the book, I feel I have connected with Assagioli at a soul level and continue to find ways to channel the essence of his being into the fabric of the work I am doing.

Acknowledgements

Most of the people I want to acknowledge in relationship to this book have been mentioned in the preface above. Foremost my thanks go to Paul Elliott for his friendship, support and the creative partnership we have enjoyed these last five years. I may have the greater capacity for writing about psychosynthesis coaching, but he has the greater gift for living and practising it. I have learned much from him which goes unrecognised and he is the silent partner in the enterprise of this book. I am in the debt of both Roger and Joan Evans for many things, not least for my four years of training at the Institute, for supporting myself and Paul in establishing Psychosynthesis Coaching Limited and for our continuing creative partnership. More recently Roger has been particularly inspirational on his recent coaching supervision course, as he continues to evolve his vision and understanding of psychospiritual coaching. Of the many others involved with the Institute who have supported our venture, I particularly want to acknowledge Anne Welsh, who has encouraged and supported us from the start, as well as Maggie Hacker, Debbie Friedman, Steve Bethnal and the others who so ably lead the Fundamentals of Psychosynthesis courses.

Then there are the many practising psychosynthesis coaches and supervisors who have contributed directly or indirectly to my being able to write this book. This includes Harriet Hanmer, Sue Cruse, Steve O'Shaughnessy and Martin Egan as the other members of my ongoing supervision training group; Gordon Symons and Ruth Rochelle as co-facilitators on our PGCPLC courses; and the group of psychosynthesis coaching MA graduates with whom I worked in various capacities over the last six years, including Martin Armitage-Smith, Matthew Burdock and John Crossan. During the writing of this book, my understanding of psychosynthesis or coaching has been enhanced enormously through meeting and exchange within an increasingly international network. In particular these include Alessandra Moretti, Maria-Bernadette Schenker, Giovanna Bratti, Raffaella di Savoia and others from the IIPE in Verona, Petra Guggisberg Nocelli whose wonderful book has been an inspiration, Isabelle

Kung, Kenneth Sorensen, Didi Firman in the US and Keith Silvester as the president of the European Federation for Psychosynthesis Psychotherapy (EFPP).

I want to thank all my clients, from whom I am sure I learned more than they did from me over the years. In writing this book, if there is anyone whose work I have drawn from inadvertently without acknowledgement, I apologise.

As already mentioned, I owe an enormous debt to our PGCPLC students, alongside whom I have been deepening my learning over the last four years. There are too many to mention by name but this seems a good place to sign-post the directory of practising psychosynthesis coaches, which can be found on our PCL website.

Most importantly I want to acknowledge my wife Diana for her love and support for the work I am engaged in. Somehow, she managed to trust me when I set out on the path that led to writing this book. I acknowledge her spiritual wisdom, which helps ground my experience of psychosynthesis, and should recognise that she set off down the psychosynthesis path long before I did and even predicted my creative partnership with Roger Evans before I knew him. Diana also edited a draft of this book, offering valuable feedback and suggestions that helped curtail the worst excesses of my writing style. Finally, I acknowledge Roberto Assagioli, whom I never met but with whom I feel a heart connection, his kind and wise spirit radiating through the many souls he touched directly as well as through his work, which continues to evolve.

Introduction and overview

As above, so below:
As within, so without.
Hermes Trismegistus

What this book is about

As the coaching profession develops, more and more coaches are looking
beyond conventional behavioural and performance-oriented coaching
approaches to ways of working at greater depth within the context of an
increasingly complex, uncertain and stressful world. Some leadership coaches
may start to find clients are taking them into emotional and personal territory
for which they do not feel adequately prepared.

This book responds to the call of coaches who want to be able to work with
the whole person, with the inner as well as the outer worlds, and not just at
rational and behavioural levels but at emotional and spiritual levels as well,
without necessarily embarking upon a lengthy psychotherapy training.

Psychosynthesis, often described as a 'psychology of Self and Will', is
unique amongst psychologies in the emphasis it places on *Self* and *Will* at
the centre of human psychological functioning. An understanding of how
to nurture and release free will and creativity within individuals has never
been more important to the profession of coaching. In this VUCA age – of
volatility, uncertainty, complexity and ambiguity – leaders often struggle
to navigate outer pressures, turbulence and change alongside inner stresses,
doubts and crises, let alone actively lead the evolutionary change that is
called for within their organisations. This book introduces psychosynthesis
coaching and shows how this holistic and integrative psychology can provide
the foundations for working with the whole person in ways that respond to
today's emergent crises.

At the outset, we need to make it clear that the coach's ability to practice this approach will depend upon their own level of personal development,
psychospiritual training and coaching experience. We help the reader assess

their own level of development and review possible options for continued personal and professional development in support of working in this way.

We show why a holistic psychological approach must include being able to navigate all levels of consciousness within the human psyche; the pre-personal (or lower unconscious) and transpersonal (or superconscious) as well as the personal (or middle unconscious and consciousness). We show why a psychological approach must be grounded by a theory or model of the *self*. We explain the key concepts and models of psychosynthesis, including the self, will and spiritual emergence, and show how these provide a solid foundation for coaches to develop psychospiritual mindedness. We elaborate the core model of psychosynthesis coaching – the context, models, methods, skills and techniques for psychosynthesis coaches to draw upon in working with their clients.

We directly tackle the issue of the boundary between therapy and coaching and show why coaches need to be able to work with pre-personal material without regressing or therapising their clients, as well as with transpersonal or psycho-spiritual material and issues. By 'transpersonal', we are referring to the domain of our higher aspirations and potential as human beings, including identity, purpose, meaning and values. We are also including the inner crises of identity, meaning or duality that many people experience at some point in their lives.

There have been many significant developments over the last decade or three, such as in developmental psychology, systemic coaching, somatic working and mindfulness practices, which can combine well with psychosynthesis. These can even be seen as developments of aspects of psychosynthesis. However, on their own, they all might suffer from not being grounded in a robust and comprehensive psychology of the whole person. We seek to bring these other perspectives together within the context and model of psychosynthesis coaching.

This book is structured according to nineteen chapters, an outline of each of which is provided below. This is also intended to give you, the reader, a sense of the overall flow of the book and enable you to read the book in the way that suits you best.

Chapter 1: Context is all

What is coaching? What is psychosynthesis coaching? How is it different from other coaching approaches?

We start with a definition of psychosynthesis coaching and describe how it is different to other coaching approaches. I introduce a dynamic practitioner framework as a more nuanced way of reflecting upon coaching practice. I then introduce the concept of coaching the *being* and how this contrasts with most coaching approaches that are concerned with coaching *doing* or behaviour.

This is set within the context of a brief overview of coaching and how it is developing as a profession. I touch upon the key distinctions in coaching: between coaching activity and the coaching profession; between life and leadership or organisational or executive coaching; between external and internal organisational coaching; between specialist coaches and leaders as coaches.

Chapter 2: Origins, elders and developments

Who was Roberto Assagioli, the founder of psychosynthesis? Who are the pioneers of psychosynthesis coaching? How has it developed since Assagioli's day?

We introduce Roberto Assagioli's life and works to the reader and provide an overview of the work of Evans, Whitmore, Firman and others who have applied psychosynthesis to meeting the emerging needs of organisational leadership and coaching. Developments and applications to the organisational world have been taking place since Assagioli's day, in particular through the work of Roger Evans and the London Institute, but also through the practice of many organisational practitioners and coaches who have been trained in psychosynthesis. I describe this work and show how it provides a foundation for further developments.

Chapters 3, 7 and 10: Personal and professional – in three parts

Why are personal and professional development inseparable in coaching? Why does this work start with you?

The coach's ability to practise this psychospiritual approach depends upon their own level of personal development, psychological training and coaching experience. In these chapters we extensively unpack the whole field of personal development, drawing upon my own personal odyssey, and help the reader assess their current level of development and review possible options for continued personal and professional development.

I am separating this massive topic into three parts and weaving it in between other chapters that carry forwards the central narrative of the book (concerning psychosynthesis and leadership and coaching), partly to make it more digestible to the reader but also to keep bringing the reader back to their own development as the cornerstone of this professional pathway.

In the first part, Chapter 3, we explain what we mean by *personal development* and how it combines with professional development for the psychosynthesis coach. In the second part, Chapter 7, we draw out seven important perspectives for coaches that show how personal and professional development are interdependent. In the third part, Chapter 10, we provide an overview of some maps and models that help us recognise our personality types, our psychological preferences or biases, and, given these, our likely edges or issues to work on.

Chapter 4: The leadership challenge and the call to coaching

What is the nature of the leadership challenge in today's organisations and society? How does psychosynthesis speak to today's crisis of leadership? In what ways is Roberto Assagioli's writing and teaching relevant and applicable to what is happening today?

We examine the challenges that leadership and leaders are facing today, how the fundamental relationship between the individual and the organisation has changed and the implications this has for coaching. The typical individual leader is facing mounting organisational challenges and performance pressures that bring corresponding personal stress and psychological pressures. The boundaries between business and personal are becoming blurred and harder to manage. More to the point, being a leader these days has a very personal dimension that needs to be recognised and supported.

We then explore the proposition that Assagioli's work brings something important to today's challenges and crises of leadership. This includes an exposition of the current crises, and draws in particular upon the Act of Will, so as to illustrate the value and relevance of Assagioli's message.

Chapter 5: Coaching psychology

Why does coaching need to be underpinned by psychology? Why does leadership coaching need a psychospiritual psychology?

To fully appreciate the value of psychosynthesis within coaching, we must first understand why coaching needs psychology in the first place and why coaches need to be psychologically minded in the way they work. Then we need to distinguish between different types of coaching psychologies and place psychosynthesis within this broader context. We argue that, given the nature of the emergent leadership crisis and the spiritual crises experienced by many leaders, a psycho-spiritual perspective is needed now more than ever. In other words, a psychology with soul has particular value for coaches wishing to work at this level.

Chapter 6: psychosynthesis as a coaching psychology

What does psychosynthesis provide as a core coaching psychology? How do key concepts of psychosynthesis, including the Will and Self, inform, guide and support leadership coaching?

Having started with the needs of leadership coaching for a psychology, I then take the perspective of psychosynthesis as an integrative and holistic psychology and show what it offers as a core coaching psychology. I describe some of the key concepts and show how they are applicable to the territory of leadership coaching. I present how psychosynthesis provides a psycho-spiritual psychology for coaches who want to want to work at the deepest level and in the most impactful way with their clients within the context of today's emergent leadership challenges.

Chapter 8: The full model of psychosynthesis coaching

What is our full model of psychosynthesis coaching? What is the context and method of psychosynthesis coaching? What are the key models, tools and skills?

From this foundation of showing why psychosynthesis works as a core coaching psychology, I fully elaborate the psychosynthesis coaching model. This starts with Roger Evans' model of trifocal vision and how we use this as both the context and primary method for *coaching the being*. Around this, I then build the other models which are needed by coaches; for example models of coaching *agendas*, coaching *process* and coaching *interventions*.

Chapter 9: Boundaries, ambiguities and contexts

What distinguishes psychosynthesis leadership coaching from life coaching? What distinguishes psychosynthesis coaching from therapy? How might leaders develop their skills as psychosynthesis coaches?

Once we have fully elaborated our model, we are able to more fully describe the scope of leadership coaching, as well as explore the boundaries and limitations of the work we can do. This includes elaborating the complexities of working with leaders in organisations and why this requires additional skills and experience to those of the life coach.

We consider how psychosynthesis coaching can be used by leaders directly in the way they work with their people and teams. We also look at how the approach works for internal coaches as contrasted with external coaches.

Chapter 11: Leadership development

How does psychosynthesis inform and support leadership development in coaching?

As we expand our perspective from individual to group and organisation and hold the individual within the context of these larger systems, we can also expand our concept of personal development to one of leadership development. I will show how and why psychosynthesis is of particular value in supporting leadership development, and how Assagioli's model of individual self-actualisation and self-realisation can be enhanced by more recent works in developmental psychology.

I take coaching into the realm of leadership development by distinguishing between horizontal, vertical and inner development, and explore the relationship between these three aspects or domains. I introduce Roger Evans' Five Dimensions of Leadership as the core model for supporting the inner development of leaders for psychosynthesis coaches.

Chapter 12: Coaching in organisational systems and the systemic perspective

How does psychosynthesis coaching work at the organisational level? How does it engage with organisational systems? How does a systemic perspective enhance our work as leadership coaches? How do we develop the capacity for systemic awareness in the leaders we coach?

Having introduced the organisational dimension of leadership coaching, in this section I expand this further by bringing in relevant psychosynthetic perspectives on the systemic nature of organisations.

We trace the origins of the systemic perspective, explore how we can work with systemic approaches in organisations and ponder the critical question of how to develop systemic awareness in our clients.

Chapter 13: The developmental perspective

How does the developmental perspective complement or augment the psychospiritual perspective? How might psychosynthesis be combined with developmental psychology and various approaches within this?

We spend some time unpacking the developmental perspective more fully and show how holding this lens is both valuable and essential for leadership coaching. I provide an overview of Wilber's integral-developmental model, as well the adult-worldview-developmental perspective based upon Laloux's organisational paradigms and Clare Graves' value systems.

We show how these developmental models also provide systemic perspectives on what is going on within ourselves, our organisations and society. We broaden and generalise the developmental view to the evolutionary perspective by exploring the shape, principle and pattern of the evolution of human consciousness, and suggest how the evolutionary spiral can be mapped onto the egg diagram map of the psyche.

Chapter 14: The somatic perspective

How might psychosynthesis be combined with somatic work and various approaches within this?

We spend some time unpacking the somatic perspective and show how working in this way brings an essential dimension to leadership coaching.

Chapter 15: Coaching leaders in change, in crisis and towards synthesis

How does the psychosynthesis coach support leaders through change? When does change become crisis? How do we support leaders through crisis? How do we support leaders to create inner and outer synthesis through working with subpersonalities and the balance of opposites? How can we or our clients engage with synthesis as a transformational path in our lives?

Much of coaching is about change, either helping clients bring about change in themselves and their lives or supporting them through periods of change and crisis. We start by unpacking the different types, levels and dimensions of change and exploring how these might come into coaching. We take the coach through how the three-phase, ten-step process of mindset change process works, followed by the psychosynthesis approach to working with subpersonalities. We then explore the complex and challenging topic of crisis and how coaches might work with clients who are experiencing different forms of crisis. Finally, we turn our attention to the process of synthesis and how coaches might help their leader clients to create synthesis through working in both the inner and outer dimensions.

Chapter 16: Coaching the Will

How does Assagioli's approach to developing the Will help leaders today? In what ways was his introspective scientific research decades ahead of today's experimental psychology and neuroscience? How might we work at greater depth to develop the will with our clients?

We then pick up on some earlier themes concerning *Will*, looking at the role of will in the existential crisis of leadership and exploring how finding and activating available will is the focus of our core method of trifocal vision. We will show how the psychosynthesis coach can work with leaders to develop their will.

Chapter 17: Psychosynthesis techniques

Which psychosynthesis techniques are most valuable for coaching? How might psychosynthesis coaches draw upon a range of techniques that they can use with their clients?

Finally, we consider how some psychosynthesis techniques might be used in coaching. The disidentification meditation is central to the personal practice of many psychosynthesis coaches and we look at how it might be introduced directly with clients. We explore how guided meditation, visualisation and other techniques can more generally be used to activate the imagination in coaching to support clients in achieving their goals. We direct the reader towards useful sources of psychosynthesis techniques and practices that the coach might draw upon. However, we caution against using techniques without adequate context and unless there is clear purpose in doing so.

Chapter 18: Insights from neuropsychology and the implications for psychosynthesis coaches

What should the psychosynthesis coach know about neuroscience? Is neuroscience telling us anything new? How do we reconcile scientific and psycho-spiritual perspectives?

The psychosynthesis coach needs to be aware of what neuroscience and neuropsychology are telling us that might be useful to leadership coaching. I have observed that many coaches have heard of neuroscience and may have picked up some useful insights or techniques which have enhanced their work, but they don't really understand where it fits in. In this chapter we present an extensive summary of what neuroscience and neuropsychology have to offer coaching, but very much from a psycho-spiritual perspective.

Chapter 19: A new synthesis and the future of psychosynthesis coaching

How is psychosynthesis coaching developing for the future? Has this book achieved a new synthesis within the umbrella of psychosynthesis coaching? What might a new synthesis look like? How can the community of psychosynthesis coaches grow and prosper?

Finally, I turn my attention outwards and forwards to where psychosynthesis coaching might be going. What direction should psychosynthesis coaching take? What can we do to support a growing community of psychosynthesis coaches?

Chapter 1

Context is all

What is coaching? What is psychosynthesis coaching? How is it different from other coaching approaches?

The coaching context

Coaching is a fast-growing and increasingly widely accepted professional activity, both within organisations – as executive, leadership or management coaching – and within society in general, as life coaching. Yet coaching is still in the early stages of development as a professional practice and discipline, without well-defined boundaries and with an immature knowledge base. Coaching is currently many different things to different people, and the scope of what we call psychosynthesis coaching is a relatively niche and undiscovered part of this.

As with any growing profession, there is naturally an ongoing battle for the high ground in terms of defining, developing and governing the profession, with different national and international bodies offering accreditation standards and structures for coaches. There are already thousands of books about coaching, with Amazon listing 2,214 books in its Coaching and Mentoring category at the time of writing. There are now many forms of coach training and educational programmes on offer to both new and experienced coaches, with at least several dozen within the UK alone. In addition, there are many national and international bodies and associations (including ICF, AC, EMCC and APECS) helping to establish and regulate the profession through accreditation, certification and standard setting. Indeed, there is something of a battle going on for the body and soul of coaching, for the high ground and the common ground, for the mainstream of practice and the niche positions. Everyone with an interest in the subject will tend to give their own definition of coaching and their view of what constitutes good professional practice.

The ICF (the most widespread international coaching body) emphasises **process** in their definition: *ICF defines coaching as partnering with clients in* *a thought-provoking and creative* **process** *that inspires them to maximize their personal and professional potential (ICF website, 2018).*

The EMCC emphasises the **purpose** of the coaching relationship in terms of *improving performance or personal development that involves applying one or more relevant methods according to standards and ethical principles... (Gray, Garvey, Lane 2016 p302).*

For the purposes of this book, I will define the scope of what I mean by coaching by highlighting these key principles.

Coaching:

- Is a supportive, enabling and empowering professional **relationship** and **activity** that honours the autonomy, resourcefulness, creativity and responsibility of the client
- is goal-, future- or outcome-oriented in **purpose**, and yet can include working with the client in the domains of past, present or future
- is usually a **one-to-one** relationship and activity between a coach and a coaching client, which takes place within a context of confidentiality and trust, although **team** coaching is also becoming more prevalent
- is appropriate for anyone who is what the psychological profession calls a **healthy neurotic** and can function in the world
- can encompass the **inner and outer dimensions** of peoples' lives and work; personal and practical aspects; psychological and behavioural perspectives; physical, emotional, mental and spiritual levels of the client's experience

In a later section, I will add to this definition in terms of what is meant more specifically by leadership and life coaching.

Gray, Garvey and Lane in *A Critical Introduction to Coaching and Mentoring* (2016, p16) make no attempt to define coaching, and instead trace its emergence from a variety of social contexts and its spread by social means, making it a strongly social activity that draws from broad intellectual frameworks. They go on to say that '*modern coaching practices are dynamic and contextual*' with roots '*in education, sport, psychology and psychotherapy*'. This describes the complexity and ambiguity of coaching well and calls for a dynamic framework which can be used to contextualise different coaching approaches and practices.

I recently developed such a **Dynamic Practitioner Framework** (Howard (2017b) that (i) identifies differences *within* coaching practice as well as *between* coaching and other professional relationships and (ii) helps coaches think critically about how they frame the work they do and reflect upon their practice. In my teaching I also refer to this as the **4Cs**:

- **Context** – what is the context of the relationship? How has it come about? What is the wider systemic context? Are other parties involved?

- **Contract** – what formal or informal goals or outcomes are the focus of the work? How is the relationship structured and what agreements are made? What is the understanding between practitioner and client?
- **Client** – what needs, issues and agendas are they bringing? What is their ego strength and stability? What is their level and depth of personal development, self-awareness and self-responsibility?
- **Capability (or Coach)** – what is the coach's level of education and training, their professional and personal development? What is their experience and level of confidence of working in different domains or dimensions or with different types of client?

This framework further breaks into two parts:

Part One: Context and **Contract** determine the nature of the professional relationship or the *container* – whether counselling or coaching, or what kind of coaching, for example life coaching within an individual or personal context or leadership coaching within an organisational context, along with a more complex multi-party contract.

Context and contracting are all-important in any practitioner relationship. We are not just saying that different types of coaching will have different contexts, but that the practitioner (i) needs to be aware and able to hold the context of the relationship and (ii) needs the skills to contract with the client (or client system) in a way that is congruent with the context. This doesn't mean that everything should be written down and formally agreed, but the practitioner and client relationship does require a level of clarity or problems may occur. Having established these principles, a distinction can be made as to how the context and contract might differ between coaching and counselling, with the coaching context being framed as forward-looking and outcome-oriented, although this can involve working across temporal dimensions, past, present and future.

I like to hold Sir John Whitmore's (2017) principles of *awareness* and *responsibility* as part of my coaching context with clients. There is something of a paradox here in that the coach can take responsibility for holding the context while the client is responsible for their own process, actions and outcomes. One thing we stress as a possible difference from counselling is that the coach doesn't need to diagnose the client's issues; rather they are helping the client reach an understanding or diagnosis for themselves with a view to finding solutions or taking actions. As psychosynthesis coaches our focus is on Self (*who is this Being most essentially, and what is emergent for them?*) and finding available Will – what small steps or actions will take the client forwards and release more will? Something we notice with counsellors making the transition to coaching is the tendency to over-psychologise and want to fully diagnose the client's issues for themselves (and therefore spend too long in sessions working on their understanding rather than that of the coachee). This doesn't mean the coach shouldn't be curious or formulate hypotheses but that they hold these lightly and leave the primary responsibility for understanding with the client.

Contracting is a major topic in itself and Peter Bluckert's *Psychological Dimensions of Executive Coaching* (2006) is a good place to start. Most coaching contracts involve regular monthly or bi-monthly meetings and work with repeatable contractual cycles (e.g. of six sessions or three months), but leadership coaching can also allow for ad-hoc meetings or calls in response to emergent situations or crises. Counselling contracts tend to involve more frequent meetings (e.g. weekly) at the practitioner's premises and be open-ended in terms of duration. But again, there are no hard and fast rules providing there is congruence across the four Cs.

Part Two: Client and **Capability** define the scope and nature of the work that can potentially take place within the professional relationship, the ***contents*** – as determined by the openness, development and availability of the client as well as the nature of the needs and issues they bring, *coupled with* the professional capability and personal capacity of the coach. Different coaches can work at a greater or lesser level of depth involving emotional, personal and psychological ground, depending upon their training, skills and experience.

The key boundary concerning the **Client** that we hold in coaching is that we only work with functioning people with sufficient ego strength. Another way of saying this is that we work with healthy neurotics who are able to function in the world (i.e. get to work, hold down relationships, pay their bills) although it is quite possible that successful leaders are suffering psychological problems or pathologies – increasingly our leader clients bring issues and crises of anxiety, stress, addiction or depression alongside their leadership development and organisational agendas. This doesn't mean we shouldn't work with them or we should pack them off to a therapist as soon as one of these issues emerges. Nor does it mean that we will work with them as a therapist would in the area of past traumas and unresolved history. The coach can help clients become aware of how past trauma and mirrors of the past are influencing or impeding their objectives and help them take responsibility for healing or resolving these. The key here is that the coach is helping the client find their own strategy and way forward to dealing with their past at the level of the pre-personal unconscious (or psychodynamic). Sometimes this can involve referral to a counsellor or therapist for specific work alongside the coaching; sometimes it involves the client working with the coach in a boundaried context (if the coach has the experience and training), as well as engagement with all manner of other personal development and therapeutic resources or solutions (e.g. group work, somatic work, systemic work, healing, retreats, etc.).

I draw from Julia Vaughan Smith's APECS paper *What has trauma got to do with coaching? Or coaching to do with trauma?* (2015, p10) to add insight into how the coach can work in relationship to past trauma:

Coaches with understanding and experience of this field (trauma and personality splits) can bring something additional to the coaching work, a greater transitional space between the inner and outer worlds, which allows for deep transformation without working directly with the traumatised self or with the past. It needs a slightly different tool kit, perhaps, particularly for those clients who are clearly under the control of their survival strategies, if they wish to address some underlying issues within the boundaries of the coaching relationship and contract.

Key distinctions in coaching

As we started out this chapter by saying, every author, professional body and training organisation offers their own definition of what coaching is, what it's for and how it should work. However, amongst all this, there does now seem to be convergence and agreement on several key distinctions.

Our primary distinction is between coaching that takes place within an *organisational* context (variously called **executive**, **leadership** or **management** coaching) and coaching within a private or *individual* context, usually called **life** coaching. Within the organisational context there is a distinction between *external* coaching (by coaches from outside an organisation) and *internal* coaching (part or full-time coaches working within an organisation) and *management* coaching (as an activity and skill set for leaders and managers).

We make a clear distinction between leadership coaching and mentoring or mentorship, which represents a growing and valuable form of supportive relationship within many organisations.

There is a further distinction between organisational coaching, with which we are concerned here, and business coaching or coaching that focuses on a particular area of expertise that the coach may bring, for example human resources, or financial, marketing or sector experience. We should also mention sports coaching as a specialised branch of coaching that is beyond the scope of this book, not least because of the debt owed to sports coaching in the origins of organisational coaching. For our purposes, sports coaching, business coaching and the broader field of mentorship are related but separate fields (i.e. distant cousins with whom we stay in touch). As with life coaching, we are not attempting to say anything specific about these fields of practice within this book, but there is nothing to say that these other types of coach cannot learn from and incorporate aspects of psychosynthesis coaching within their practice.

This leads into the notion of hybrid coaching practice, where specific coaches may combine leadership coaching or life coaching with another form or modality of professional practice, based upon their specific history, experience, training and qualifications.

How is psychosynthesis coaching different?

Having set out this contextual frame of reference with regard to coaching, I will now turn to the question of how psychosynthesis coaching might be distinguished from other approaches to coaching. Psychosynthesis is a psychospiritual psychology, developed by Roberto Assagioli, that has been primarily applied to the field of psychotherapy – although it is also studied as a psychology in its own right and informs the wider field of personal development in a multitude of ways. As mentioned in the introduction, different forms or versions of psychosynthesis coaching have been practised for many years, some more explicitly than others, and developments have been shared continuously, both formally and informally, within the wider community of practice. Since the mid 2000s, when the Institute started offering the MA in Psychosynthesis Coaching, the development of psychosynthesis coaching has gained greater momentum under Roger Evans' leadership and with the establishment of our Post-Graduate Certificate in Psychosynthesis Leadership Coaching (PGCPLC) in 2015. The following broad context and principles help define or distinguish psychosynthesis coaching from other approaches, whilst at the same time acknowledging some diversity in practice:

> The overarching context of psychosynthesis coaching is that we are working at the level of the being and beyond the mind. We are coaching the Being/Self.

I summarised the essence of this from a recent seminar with Roger Evans. Psychosynthesis coaching is about:

- Holding a psycho-spiritual context *beyond the mind*
- Learning how to use your *heart* as the resonator of Self
- Self being witnessed by the coach – thus evoking the Self for the coachee
- Enabling the Will of the Self of the coachee to be expressed, to start acting
- …using trifocal vision and the six-session model

Roger Evans (Seminar, 14th November 2017)

We fully explain trifocal vision and the six-session model as the core model for psychosynthesis coaching in chapter eight. Some of the above bullets may appear somewhat cryptic or vague on first reading, but hopefully their meaning will become clearer as you practise and reflect upon them over time.

For now, to the above I would add these principles:

- Psychosynthesis coaching goes beyond conventional performance and behaviourally oriented approaches to work at the level of Being and what this means in the context of leadership for the client.

- Psychosynthesis coaches work with Self and Will alongside engagement with the issues, agendas and goals that the client brings to coaching.
- Psychosynthesis coaching is holistic and embraces both the inner and outer worlds of the client, according to the needs and agenda of our clients.
- Psychosynthesis coaches work with inner life issues of identity, purpose, meaning, values and crisis in their coaching practice with leaders.

Some of the above is easy to say, but not so easy to do (or to be!). Much of the rest of this book will break this down further, unpack how this works from different perspectives and look at how we go about putting it into practice.

Chapter 2

Origins, elders and developments

Who was Roberto Assagioli, the founder of psychosynthesis? Who are the pioneers of psychosynthesis coaching? How has it developed since Assagioli's day?

Roberto Assagioli, the founder of psychosynthesis

How to introduce Roberto Assagioli to someone who is new to psychosynthesis? A contemporary of Sigmund Freud, Carl Jung and later Abraham Maslow, we can emphasise his place in the history of the development of psychology in the 20th century. We can focus on his work and in particular his unfolding development of psychosynthesis over many decades. We can also try to convey the essence of who he was as a man, providing an insight into the nature and being of this remarkable person. This is probably best achieved by listening to people who knew and worked with him. A recent documentary film, *The Scientist of the Spirit,* by Maria Erica Pacileo and Fernando Maraghini, does this very well, with a mixture of commentary, talking heads and evocative images, spoken in Italian with English subtitles. I was delighted to spend some time recently with Isabelle Kung, who was interviewed in this film about her experience of spending her summers as a young woman in the company of Assagioli. Kung's eyes light up whenever she speaks about Assagioli.

Two recently published books about psychosynthesis include biographies of Roberto Assagioli which bring us close to the character of the man, as well as telling the story of his life and work. The first and most extensive is Petra Guggisberg Nocelli's beautifully written *The Way of Psychosynthesis,* describing itself as a complete guide to the field's origins, concepts and fundamental experiences, with a biography of Roberto Assagioli. This is an impressively researched book which might now claim to offer the most comprehensive and up-to-date background source for both psychosynthesis and Roberto Assagioli.

Towards the end of the biography (page 68), Nocelli summarises her impressions from interviews with those who knew Assagioli:

Everyone interviewed describes Assagioli as a simple and serene man who managed to maintain these qualities even in the most difficult and painful moments of his life... It was the simplicity of one who reached the wisdom and breadth of extraordinary vision; the simplicity of one who had made synthesis the guiding star of his whole life.

She continues:

According to those that met him, he totally embodied his message... he transformed by example, with just his presence, wordlessly and above all without imposing his ideas.

She goes on:

He could touch the soul of people. Being in contact with him transformed one, psychologically and spiritually. This, according to the interviewees, together with joy and sense of humour were his main traits. They said that after getting to know him, they were no longer the same, not so much by what he was saying but how he was.

Why are these impressions about Assagioli important? They not only illustrate authenticity and congruence with his ideas in the way he lived his life but point towards the importance of *being* within the psychology of psychosynthesis. We can sense the possibility of a truly holistic approach that encompasses all of ourselves – body, heart, mind and spirit – and that is expressed through all of who we are, how we are and what we do. For me, he is one of the few great historical thinkers whose lived example can be seen to be wholly consistent and congruent with his ideas and teaching.

Kenneth Sorensen's previously published *The Soul of Psychosynthesis* (2016), which tackles similar territory but with a different style, also includes a biography in the appendices. This is shorter and perhaps easier to read, and ends with a summation by Piero Ferrucci (one of Assagioli's students and collaborators). Within the biography (p155), Sorensen describes Assagioli's fundamental worldview as one that:

...includes both the individual and society, with a focus on synthesis and unification rather than analysis and splitting into smaller parts. Assagioli attempts to create a psychology with synthesis between Eastern mysticism and philosophy and Western psychoanalysis and logic. It was important to Assagioli that psychosynthesis remained scientific.

This captures an essential quality of psychosynthesis and points to why it is becoming increasingly relevant to the challenges and crises we are facing in society today. I will return to develop this theme on more than one occasion later in the book.

I don't want to repeat what has been done very well elsewhere but for now I will briefly summarise Assagioli's life story, using an edited version of a script used in seminars at the Institute of Psychosynthesis.

Roberto Assagioli (1888–1974) – summary of his life (edited, courtesy of The Institute of Psychosynthesis)

Born in Venice in 1888, Roberto moved in 1904 to Florence, where he spent most of the rest of his life, and died in 1974, aged 86. He lived a long life in a century of intellectual creativity and social turmoil.

He began his medical career in 1910, specialising in neurology and psychiatry, and trained with Bleuer, a colleague of Freud. After training, he started practising as a psychiatrist in Italy.

At the time Jung was working in Zurich, looking at the links between unconscious material and religious and spiritual experience. He deepened his research into the unconscious and explored the universal or, as he called it, the collective unconscious. Freud and Jung were collaborating on their theories when Freud wrote to Jung about a brilliant young psychiatrist in Florence whom he hoped would introduce psychoanalysis to Italy. Assagioli was engaged in writing a paper on their joint work.

But, as early as 1911, as Assagioli went further into developing the concepts of his own psychology, he began to feel that Freud's theory was too limited in its vision of mankind – although he did respect and took on board many of Freud's ideas on the unconscious. When his own paper came out, it was a critique of Freud's psychoanalysis; in fact, as we know, Freud and Jung eventually split over Jung's belief that the libido (our human life energy) consisted of more than sexual energy and included the impulse to spirituality as well.

So how did Assagioli come by such a different perspective, or world view, to Freud's?

Assagioli came from a cultured middle-class Jewish family background with an interest in music, art and literature. With three languages spoken in the home and throughout his childhood, Assagioli developed a passion for languages; he learned several more, including Sanskrit.

His mother was a Theosophist and he married Nella, also a Theosophist, in 1922. It was she who kindled his interest in Eastern philosophies and the esoteric mysteries – the esoteric component of his interests remaining a secret to the world, for he was also a follower of Alice Bailey and at that time such things were not generally accepted.

Assagioli's esoteric material is still to be found in the attic at his house in Florence.

He had eclectic interests from the start, and throughout his life used material from an enormous range of disciplines and interests, consistent with the flourishing growth of new knowledge in different fields at the time. His philosophy also had roots in many Eastern and Western traditions.

He loved to travel and it was his experience of meeting people from different countries and cultural backgrounds which convinced him that, at heart, human beings are the same no matter what our background and that deep down in everybody is a desire to develop to one's highest potential.

As a result of his keen interest in philosophy and culture, Assagioli became involved in various groups of liberalists and creative thinkers. Friends and contemporaries included Carl Jung, Viktor Frankl and Abraham Maslow.

Assagioli wanted to build a scientific psychology which encompassed the whole of man's potential – his creativity and will, joy and wisdom as well as the impulses and drives. In 1926, Assagioli set up the Institute of Psychosynthesis in Florence suggesting in his teaching that, at the core of the human psyche, was a spiritual self. In 1933 he presented his model of the human psyche, the egg diagram, for the first time. In spite of his theoretical interests, Assagioli saw the psychology he was evolving not merely as an abstract doctrine but as a practical path for daily living.

During the war, Assagioli was briefly imprisoned for his ideas and then, following his release, was forced into hiding from the Nazis in remote countryside, through the help of influential friends, until the end of the war. After hostilities ended, psychosynthesis started to be known internationally and Assagioli became linked with the Human Potential Movement, alongside Maslow; the two of them took Jung's transpersonal psychology to a different platform. Assagioli wrote hundreds of papers in English and Italian* and published two books: *Psychosynthesis* (1965) and *The Act of Will* (1974, just before his death. A third book, drawing together his articles on *Transpersonal Development,* was published posthumously (1986).

In 1972, a training programme was set up at the Psychosynthesis Institute in Esalen, San Francisco. The programme was received as revolutionary at the time as it encompassed both the suffering and traumas of the past (prepersonal) and the spiritual dimensions of human experience (transpersonal). Psychosynthesis started as a self-development model and was adapted for psychotherapy training over time.

Reproduced by kind permission of the Institute of Psychosynthesis, London 2020

* *Many of these have been translated into several languages, but even more are still to be published or translated – although this task is gradually being undertaken by dedicated volunteers in support of the Florence Istituto Psicosintesi – Casa Assagioli .*

Psychosynthesis – psychology or philosophy?

There is an interesting question about whether psychosynthesis is not only a psychology but also a philosophy. It might be seen as both, and can also be taken as either. However, Assagioli was careful to keep his work of developing psychosynthesis as a psychology separate from his interest and work in spirituality, mysticism and religion. Indeed, in his house in Florence, he kept his work concerning these two areas in separate places – psychology and psychiatry in his office and mystical and spiritual work in the attic room.

To quote Sorensen (2016, p161):

It was important to Assagioli that Psychosynthesis was viewed as an open psychological system in continuous development rather than a religious or philosophical doctrine. In his first book Psychosynthesis he writes "Psychosynthesis does not aim nor attempt to give a metaphysical or a theological explanation of the great Mystery – it leads to the door, but stops there."

(p5)

We could well ask, however, where does a psychospiritual psychology end and a philosophy or a spiritual practice begin? The border with spiritual practice and religion is clear and it is important that the psychospiritual psychology is kept spiritually neutral. Philosophy is the term that is most ambiguous in this context and I would suggest it can be taken in a more or less formal sense – for example as Philosophy with a small or large P. Assagioli didn't want psychosynthesis to be considered as a formal philosophy, and yet, if you engage extensively with psychosynthesis, it is difficult not to become imbued with something of a philosophy of life, at least in a loose sense, even without exploring its philosophical underpinnings.

I would suggest that as a loose philosophy it is flexible and individual: anyone can form their own unique view and experience of what psychosynthesis means as a philosophy of life. There is enough dynamic freedom within psychosynthesis as an informal philosophy to combine easily and fruitfully with other philosophies or spiritual practices. Certainly, for the purposes of this book, my concern with Psychosynthesis is as a psychospiritual psychology that can be applied broadly to personal development and, specifically, to the professional field of coaching; in other words, as a core coaching psychology.

For the reader who would like to find out more about Assagioli and psychosynthesis, I would recommend reading the books by Petra Guggisberg Nocelli and Kenneth Sorensen, cited earlier. If your interest extends beyond reading, the next step might be to attend an open day or evening at one of the training schools (the Institute or the Psychosynthesis Trust in the United Kingdom). Following that, you could attend one of the short introductory courses, usually four days long, run by the Institute or Trust. Different pathways are then open for personal development and professional training, depending upon your purpose and interest, including our own five-month Post-Graduate Certificate in Psychosynthesis Leadership Coaching.

The history of psychosynthesis coaching

For now, though, we are going to focus on the story of how psychosynthesis has become a coaching psychology. Ongoing developments and applications to coaching, leadership and the organisational world have been taking place since Assagioli's day, in particular through the work of Roger Evans and the London Institute, but also through the practice of many organisational practitioners and coaches who have been trained in psychosynthesis. In this section I attempt to do justice to the depth and breadth of this work and show how it provides a foundation for further developments.

As previously described, at least three different versions of psychosynthesis coaching have emerged: (i) Roger Evans has been developing and practising his coaching approach for many decades and the London Institute of Psychosynthesis has been training psychosynthesis coaches for more than a decade, culminating in the MA in Psychosynthesis Organisational and Leadership Coaching; (ii) Didi Firman and the Synthesis Center have been providing psychosynthesis life coach training for many years in the USA; and (iii) Sir John Whitmore referred increasingly explicitly to psychosynthesis coaching in each edition of his book *Coaching for Performance* (e.g. Part IV, 4th Edition 2009), and included this perspective in both short courses and the Masters coaching programmes he was involved in.

Below I give a little bit more background on each of these. I should acknowledge that I tend to give prominence to Roger Evans' work and the London Institute's version as our starting point in this book – primarily because this was the approach that I was trained in and also because, with trifocal vision, it provides a coherent and explicit model for psychosynthesis coaching that I have chosen to build upon.

Sir John Whitmore and Coaching for Performance

Sir John Whitmore (who died in September 2017 aged 82) played a leading role in shaping and developing the modern coaching profession. His book *Coaching for Performance*, first published in 1992, is still probably the most widely read (with more than one million copies sold) and frequently referenced book on coaching. He is also an important figure for psychosynthesis coaching because he recognised the potential role it could play, and pointed coaches who wanted to work at greater depth towards a training in psychosynthesis. Although not formally trained in psychosynthesis himself, he was married to Diana Whitmore, who founded and led the Psychosynthesis and Education Trust in London. Diana also authored Psychosynthesis Counselling in Action (originally 1991, second edition 2000), one of the key texts for counsellors, which offers much of value for coaches too.

Although the main thrust of John Whitmore's seminal book *Coaching for Performance* is about performance coaching using the GROW model (see Chapter 8 in this book), in the later editions he starts to include a broader view of coaching and explicitly lays the ground for psychosynthesis coaching. In the fourth edition (2009) he adds a whole section on 'Transformation through Transpersonal Coaching", in which he discusses the importance of emotional intelligence in leadership, introduces spiritual intelligence and starts to lay the ground for coaches working with leaders experiencing crises of purpose, meaning and values. He goes on to say (p204):

> So how does a coach work with such issues and what skills does he or she need? Certainly, to be most effective coaches do need to go beyond the basic skill level of asking questions to raise awareness and responsibility, listening well, running the coachee's agenda and following the GROW sequence. There is much more to coaching than that and this takes us into the next evolution of psychology.

He then describes how he was drawn to psychosynthesis as a 'whole system perspective of psychology' that 'has informed my coaching ever since'. He goes on (p206) to describe how:

> Psychosynthesis offers a number of maps and models, the strands of which weave a very useful cradle for in-depth coaching. One of these is a simplified model of human development that, like all models, is not the truth but merely a representation that enables a conversation to take place with a coach or within our own minds. A psychosynthesis-trained coach will invite the coachee to reframe life as a developmental journey. To see the creative potential within each problem, to see obstacles as stepping stones, and to imagine that we all have a purpose in life with challenges and obstacles to overcome in order to fulfil that purpose.

Whitmore goes on to outline the psychosynthesis *two-dimensions of growth model* (i.e. Assagioli's self-actualisation and self-realisation, which is explained in the next chapter), and explore how the coach can draw upon subpersonalities as well as other psychosynthesis models and tools. He also introduces Assagioli's egg diagram as a way for coaches to develop a deeper understanding of the human psyche. He touches upon working with leaders who are experiencing crisis, but explains (p210):

> I will not go into more detail here about the techniques and potential pitfalls of coaching people through a major crisis of meaning once it happens. It can be a profound experience and an unsettling time for people who have travelled a long way along the horizontal plane before it occurs. I strongly advocate some training in psychosynthesis or a similar psychology for independent coaches who wish to enter this field or may unexpectedly find themselves there.

Although some of the above is repeated in the latest fifth edition within a newly shaped chapter on 'Advanced Coaching', I have stuck with quoting the fourth edition as it presents the clearest call by Whitmore for psychosynthesis coaching. John Whitmore and Hetty Einzig (a long-time colleague and collaborator of his at Performance Consultants International, who is trained in psychosynthesis psychotherapy) co-authored a chapter on transpersonal coaching (chapter 9 in *Excellence in Coaching: the industry guide*, 2015) which introduces readers to many of the tools and techniques of psychosynthesis for coaching. Their organisation still offers two-day introductions to psychosynthesis coaching following this approach.

Performance Consultants International and The Performance Coach (with whom Diana Whitmore has been a director and part of the faculty for many years) were also involved in setting up the first Masters-level programme in coaching: the MSc in Coaching and Development, in partnership with the University of Portsmouth, which included transpersonal modules taught by Diana Whitmore and Hetty Einzig. Einzig recently wrote *The Future of Coaching: Vision, Leadership and Responsibility in a Transforming World* (2017), which provides some fascinating broader perspectives on the relevance of transpersonal coaching.

We can all be enormously appreciative of the work done by Sir John Whitmore and his colleagues to progress the cause of psychosynthesis within coaching, but at the same time be aware of its limits. What do I mean by this? Firstly, *Performance Coaching* is written in a clear, introductory and practical style that makes it accessible to mainstream audiences in leadership and coaching and helps explain its popularity. Whitmore is extremely good at making what might otherwise be seen as non-mainstream ideas (i.e. psychological and spiritual ideas) both simple and relevant in the context of today's organisational world. His intended audience includes managers, leaders and coaches who are new to the concept of coaching rather than coaches who are seeking to deepen and develop their practice. Whitmore recognises and touches upon depth without going to the depth.

Secondly, in writing about psychosynthesis, Whitmore and Einzig's emphasis is on the models, tools and techniques that it brings to modern performance coaching. As will become clearer, the approach pioneered by Roger Evans which I am developing in this book looks to create a different set of foundations for coaching, placing more emphasis on working at psychological depth with Self and Will. Whitmore and Einzig describe psychosynthesis as a transpersonal psychology, whereas we see it as a psychospiritual psychology – the importance of this distinction will become clear later.

Thirdly, Whitmore describes transpersonal or psychosynthesis coaching as a specialisation, whereas we seek to build a new conception of psychosynthesis coaching which is relevant to all leadership coaching, albeit adapted to the leader's level of development, their self-awareness and the presenting issues and agendas. However, we all agree that psychosynthesis coaching is an advanced form of coaching that builds upon the basic skills and development of the coach as described by Whitmore above (p204 quote).

Life coaching in North America

In 2018 Dorothy (Didi) Firman edited and published *The Call of Self: Psychosynthesis Life Coaching*, through the Synthesis Center Press, involving no less than 30 contributors, including myself and Roger Evans. Although there are some European contributors like us, most are from North America, and the book illustrates and celebrates the dynamic and diverse growth of psychosynthesis life coaching in America within which Didi Firman and the Synthesis Center has played a central role for more than 40 years. Didi was the founder of the Synthesis Center, which has been running a psychosynthesis life coach certification program for 20 years, alongside which Didi now plays an advisory role to the many other life coach training programs that have grown out from this base, for example Jon Schottland's certification program in New Hampshire. In her biography, Didi describes how she has been practising psychosynthesis her entire adult life, has been a psychotherapist and is a retired professor of psychology, before hinting at a gradual retirement that involves occasional workshops and training, some coaching and coaching supervision. In the editor's note to Chapter 3 of *The Call of Self*, Didi describes the legacy to life coaching in the Americas left by Martha Crampton, a student of Roberto Assagioli, and how she was Didi's primary psychosynthesis teacher and a valued mentor. The article 'Empowerment of the Will through Life Coaching', written in 2000, represents our earliest psychosynthesis orientation to the field of coaching. Sadly, Crampton died in 2009.

I recommend reading or at least dipping into *The Call of Self: Psychosynthesis Life Coaching* (2018) to anyone who wants to broaden and deepen their understanding of psychosynthesis coaching or who has a specific interest in life coaching. However, it is important to point out that these two books are doing different things. A key distinction is my focus on leadership coaching rather than life coaching; another is that, as the sole author of this book, I am seeking to provide the reader with a cohesive and comprehensive approach to psychosynthesis coaching – contrasting with the diversity and different approaches that can be found within *The Call of Self*. I hope readers will find the two works to be complementary.

Roger Evans and the London Institute of Psychosynthesis

Alongside directing and teaching at the London Institute of Psychosynthesis, which he co-founded more than 40 years ago with his wife Joan (both having studied with Assagioli before his death), Roger has run his own boutique consulting and coaching company, Creative Leadership Consultants (CLC). When I completed my four-year training with the Institute in 2004, Roger invited me to join his team of psychosynthesis-trained consultants and coaches as an associate, working mostly on projects for large complex organisations (e.g. in pharmaceuticals, financial services, infrastructure projects) going through significant change (e.g. mergers and acquisitions, transformational change programmes, downsizing) and involving coaching senior leaders and their teams. Often these projects would lead into secondary engagements with the leaders we were working with, for example involving team and leadership development. I worked with Roger and CLC on several such projects over the following decade, including a relationship with one medium-sized pharma over six years (2007–2013), which I have written about elsewhere (Howard, 2016). This represented a rich period or learning for me about how to coach senior leaders and their teams, applying my psychosynthesis training in practice and building upon my learning from the MSc in Change Agent Skills and Strategies with the Human Potential Research Group (HPRG) at Surrey University in the 1990s. This was also the highly creative period during which our current approach to psychosynthesis coaching really started to take shape, and Roger evolved his two core models for leadership coaching – Trifocal vision and the Five Dimensions of Leadership. The full story of how this happened is too long to tell here and, in any case, Roger has told his version in his recently published *5DL – The Five Dimensions of Leadership* (2020).

When I attended the 40th anniversary celebrations for the London Institute of Psychosynthesis in September 2013, I was struck by a thought about Roger and his work which I haven't shared widely before now. It seemed to me that there were really (at least) two distinct 'Rogers' – the Institute Roger working psycho-spiritually with students and the CLC Roger working with senior leaders and their organisations from more psychological, systemic and pragmatic perspectives. I wondered how well these two Rogers really knew each other and what might happen if they became better acquainted. My experience of working in partnership with Roger over the subsequent five years to set up Psychosynthesis Coaching Limited and run our PGCPLC courses, and also as a student/colleague on his PGC in psychosynthesis coaching supervision, is that somehow this has happened, coinciding with a further evolution of trifocal vision as his core model of psychosynthesis coaching. I also now experience a continuing evolution of psychosynthesis coaching taking place in the space between all the various courses and programmes we are running and with the broader psychosynthesis coaching community. This is so much so that, even since I started writing this book, whole new layers of insight have emerged.

Where does Roger's approach depart from what has come before? How does it differ from that of John Whitmore and the tradition of life coaching in North America in particular? Although the full answer will come from reading this book, let me summarise some key points. As touched upon above, this approach is primarily about how the coach works with the Self and Will of the coachee, rather than about how to use psychosynthesis models, tools and techniques in coaching (which we come to later).

This is about the nature and experience of *being* within the coaching relationship and, as a coach, how to bring our whole selves to working with the whole self of the other. This concept involves an essential shift from a psychological to a psychospiritual approach, working beyond the concrete mind at the level of being. There is also a much greater emphasis on working with the Will in Roger's approach than I have seen elsewhere and a very practical approach to how to release, activate and develop the will of the coachee. Roger also brings a very explicit systemic perspective to coaching which I have not found so apparent elsewhere. There are further distinctions and developments which have come through our own work at Psychosynthesis Coaching which I will introduce throughout the book, but for now that introduces Roger's works and contribution to psychosynthesis coaching and completes this background-building chapter.

Chapter 3

Personal and professional

Part I

'The unexamined life is not worth living...' Socrates as reported by Plato

Part I: personal development and the leadership coach

Most coaching approaches will put some attention on personal development for the coach. Sometimes this is given little more than lip service; in other cases it represents a more serious commitment. It is interesting to note that APECS is unique amongst the coaching professional bodies in asking potential members to describe their previous development in terms of professional and *personal* development (which they term CPPD).

Psychosynthesis coaching involves working with the inner as well as the outer world of our clients whilst holding a developmental context alongside other agendas and goals. The inner world concerns much more than our everyday awareness: it comprises our interior lives of thoughts and feelings, hopes and fears, dreams and anxieties; our light and our shadow and the heights and depths of our unconscious. The territory includes working with the psyche and the Self in all its dimensions, which we will describe more fully in Chapter 6. Within this context, personal development is both essential and central to the development of the coach and their professional practice. Personal development isn't an add-on or optional extra to professional development; it is what makes coaching in this way at deeper levels possible and increases our capacity to do it well. In this chapter we will show why this is the case and explore what we mean by personal development in this context.

Of course, the nature of human development and how we work with it in coaching is a recurring theme in this book. In Chapter 11 we focus more specifically on leadership development and introduce a framework that distinguishes the dimensions of horizontal, vertical and inner development. In Chapter 13 we explore more fully how human development takes place at individual and collective levels, drawing upon various developmental theories and models. But before we start to look in these later chapters at how development takes place and how to facilitate it for others, I am inviting you as the reader to take a closer look at your relationship with your own development and to challenge you to reflect upon it in new ways. I will go further and suggest that it would be fairly pointless to learn about psychosynthesis coaching as an approach which encompasses various methods, models, tools and skills without continuously drawing upon yourself and your own experience of development as an inner reference point.

Psychosynthesis can itself be described as an holistic approach to personal development, involving what Roberto Assagioli called *personal* and *transpersonal* psychosynthesis, as we follow our individual journeys towards self-realisation and self-actualisation. Following a brief introduction to the topic of personal development, I will expand upon this psychosynthesis context with specific reference to Assagioli's work.

What is personal development?

Personal development is a vast and complex topic that can be approached in many different ways. It is interwoven with the whole field of psychology, the story of the human potential movement, the leadership and talent development world, the popular self-help industry and of course the modern coaching profession. You are likely to have your own understanding of what personal development is, based upon your history and experience, so whatever your starting point and whatever perspectives you bring are valid and relevant to the theme we are exploring here.

I choose the work of Abraham Maslow and his concepts of self-actualisation and the hierarchy of needs as a useful starting point for defining personal development, not least because many others have done so before me.

As early as 1943 Maslow defined self-actualisation (p383) as '… *the desire to become more and more what one is, to become everything that one is capable of becoming* '. Adding to this, the Skills You Need website (www.skillsyouneed. com) says:

> Self-actualisation refers to the desire that everybody has 'to become everything that they are capable of becoming'. In other words, it refers to self-fulfilment and the need to reach full potential as a unique human being. Maslow also says (1970, p.383) that all individuals have the need to see themselves as competent and autonomous, also that every person has limitless room for growth.

This website then offers a number of practical steps and resources for creating your vision, planning, starting, recording and reviewing your personal development. This is certainly a useful introduction to the discipline of personal development for many people working in organisations.

In an online blog post, Myrko Thum defines personal development as '*the conscious pursuit of personal growth by expanding self-awareness and knowledge and improving personal skills'* and quotes Jung: *'until you make the unconscious conscious, it will direct your life and you will call it fate'*, as a way to focus personal development on working with the unconscious. He goes on to cite the well-known 'four stages of competence' model (first articulated by Martin Broadwell in 1969) – where we start in unconscious incompetence in our relationship to a skill or capability (*it's not on our radar*), then move to conscious incompetence as we recognise the need to develop the capability (*we want to be able to do it*), eventually build our conscious competency (*we can do it but we need to think about it*) before this becomes habit and part of our unconscious competence (*we do it automatically*). I have often seen trainers explaining this sequence using the example of learning to drive to illustrate the stages, but really it can be applied to anything, including coaching skills and models.

Another well-known tool for working with the conscious and unconscious in relation to personal development is the **Johari Window** (see Figure 3.1), created by psychologists Joseph Luft (1916–2014) and Harrington Ingham (1916–1995) in 1955 as a model that helps people better understand their relationship with themselves and others (Luft, 1963, 1969). A simple four-quadrant grid is created by combining what is *known to self* and *unknown to self* on one (X) axis, and what is *known to others* and *not known to others* along the other (Y) axis. This creates four 'windows' (or 'rooms' as Charles Handy used to say), namely the **open** space, the **hidden** area, the **blind** spot and the **unknown**. The objective in terms of improving relationship with others is to maximise the size of the open arena through exercising the key skills of appropriate **self-disclosure** (to reduce our hidden area) and asking for and receiving **feedback** (to reduce our blind spot area). Of course, this is easier said than done and takes a lifetime of practice, but it represents another

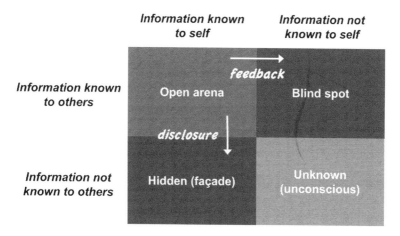

Figure 3.1 The Johari window: created by Joseph Luft and Harrington Ingham.

useful starting point for engaging in personal development alongside team and organisational development.

When I first encountered this model in the 1990s, I was always curious about how we might explore the unknown or unconscious area more fully and was never very satisfied with the answers I received at the time. Whilst pursuing other avenues of enquiry, this led me to study psychosynthesis, which seemed unique in providing a holistic map of the psyche that can help us recognise and navigate all the dimensions of our consciousness and unconsciousness, including what is sometimes called the shadow. To quote Robert Bly (1988, p1), *'"Shadow" is one of Carl Jung's most useful terms for a part of the human psyche… it conveys a visual image – we might call the shadow "the dark, unlit and repressed side of the ego complex"'*.

My own conception of personal development is that it concerns the continuing development of the *person*, the *whole human being*, or our *personhood*, however we might say it. Personal development is loosely synonymous with self-development and personal growth, although as a term it is now most commonly used to refer to the discipline, practice and professional field of working on ourselves. It is important to remember here that this practice is always owned by ourselves, by the individual, and that we alone hold agency and responsibility for it. I cannot have a personal development objective for you, only for myself, although I can support you in your personal development, as we do as coaches.

The implication here is that we need a theory or model of the person, of the whole human being, as a reference point for personal development. Without this, different approaches tend to work unconsciously from a received set of assumptions about the psyche that have not been made explicit. Psychosynthesis offers such a model, as well as a more nuanced understanding of where personal development might take us, and this is where I will now turn.

A brief aside – we are using the word *personal* in several different ways, which may cause some confusion. As well as meaning *of the person*, as described above, it also conveys the meaning of *individual*, so when we refer to personal development we are really referring to our unique individual development (as opposed to team or organisational development). Within this broad sense of the person, we focus on the *personality*, as with the use of personality profiling tools and addressing personality edges and issues. Finally, within psychosynthesis we are using *personal* to describe the *middle* or most accessible realm of the human consciousness, as opposed to the *lower* unconscious or prepersonal, or the *higher* unconscious or transpersonal. *Personal* can also be used to mean the private (or possibly off-limits in leadership coaching) aspect of our lives (as contrasted with business-personal), but we are not drawing upon that meaning here. Phew, this can be complicated!

Psychosynthesis as a path for personal development

The relationship between Maslow's and Assagioli's work and how they informed each other is a recurring topic in my writing. Assagioli recognised 'that people are not equally developed from the psychological and spiritual point of view' (1991, p107) and offers a way of understanding how personal development takes place along two interrelated but distinct dimensions. He recognised and endorsed Maslow's work concerning self-actualisation but showed how this only takes us so far in terms of understanding how people develop and grow psycho-spiritually.

Drawing upon his map of the psyche (the egg diagram), which distinguishes between prepersonal, personal and transpersonal levels of consciousness (see here), Assagioli distinguishes two dimensions of development (1974, p121; see Figure 3.2):

> In the terminology of psychosynthesis, self-actualization corresponds to personal psychosynthesis. This includes the development and harmonizing of all human functions and potentialities at all levels of the lower and middle area in the diagram of the constitution of man. Instead, self-realization concerns the third higher level, that of the superconscious, and pertains to transpersonal or spiritual psychosynthesis.

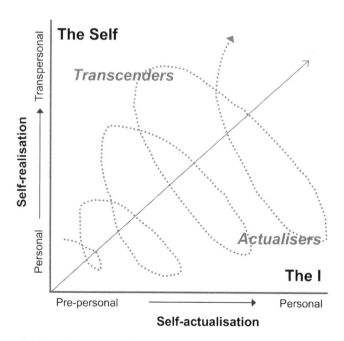

Figure 3.2 Two dimensions of self-development.

Maslow's later work recognised this distinction as he started to speak in terms of transcending self-actualisers as well as non-transcending self-actualisers. Assagioli's model of individual self-actualisation and self-realisation is our orienting model for psychosynthesis coaching in relationship to personal development. There has been much debate within the psychosynthesis world about the relationship between the two dimensions of development: whether they are sequential (personal psychosynthesis broadly preceding transpersonal psychosynthesis), concurrent (we are working on both aspects much of the time) or follow a pattern that is unique to each individual (which I tend to favour). In the graphic above I have drawn a spiral as an example of the way we might illustrate a personal journey alternating between the two dimensions.

The important thing here is that this model helps us hold the tension between self-actualisation and self-realisation and be curious about the developmental journey of ourselves and our clients. For example some of us might lean towards self-realisation (transcenders) and others towards self-actualisation (actualisers) in our personal development journey. This gives us a clue as to the type of challenges and crises we might encounter along the way. Transcenders tend to encounter crises of *duality* as they struggle with embodiment, with being spirit in matter, with making their way in the world and dealing with the practicalities of life. Actualisers tend to encounter crises of *meaning* as they strive to achieve and succeed, often evoking considerable stress in pursuit of actualising their potential in the world. Some of us will recognise both states from reflecting upon different periods of our life, and we might start to trace a pattern which resembles the spiral above (see my example below).

The focus of *personal psychosynthesis* is on developing a strong and healthy personal 'I' (sometimes referred to the I-self, small self or the personality), as the centre of our everyday awareness and self-consciousness, the psychological container and vehicle through which we experience our higher Self and actualise our potential in our lives through engaging our will. This is about being able to function happily and effectively as human beings, both in our inner experiential lives and our outer lives of relationships and actions. This part of personal development is about working on ourselves and our personality edges, blind spots and distortions that are unwelcomed and unconscious echoes of the past. The key here is to build a level of self-awareness, knowledge and acceptance that gives us sufficient psychological and behavioural freedom to activate our will, rather than necessarily changing the way we are, which is not always possible or even desirable!

The focus of *transpersonal* psychosynthesis is on the Self – who we are most essentially, the source of our being and our becoming. Without getting too technical about this more spiritual domain, we are talking here about all the ancient and modern paths to self-realisation, self-discovery or enlightenment. This part of personal development is about learning to listen to, resonate with, reach towards and recognise our essential being and unrealised potential. This is particularly difficult because most of the time we are too identified with different parts of our experience, personality or outer lives to be able to listen to the Self. Hence the need to start with personal psychosynthesis and the practice of disidentification and identification. This work is about discovering meaning and purpose for our lives from within rather than externally.

I want to explain some more about what Assagioli meant by self-realisation in this psycho-spiritual context. In the box below I have summarised his thinking from his work as published in 1965 (some of the language is a little arcane and something may have been lost in translation):

Roberto Assagioli, from Psychosynthesis (1965, p21–22) – summary:

The stages for the attainment of this goal (of self-realisation):

1. Thorough knowledge of one's personality
2. Control of its various elements
3. Realisation of one's true Self – the discovery or creation of a unifying centre
4. Psychosynthesis – the formation or reconstruction of the personality around the new centre

We have recognised that in order really to know ourselves... it is not enough to make an inventory of the elements that form our conscious being... an extensive exploration of the vast regions of our unconscious must also be undertaken.

We have first to penetrate courageously into the pit of our **lower unconscious** in order to discover the dark forces that ensnare and menace us... (e.g. by the use of the methods of psychoanalysis... and this is accomplished more easily with the help of another).

Psychoanalysis generally stops here, but this limitation is not justified. The regions of the **middle** and **higher unconscious** should also be explored. In that way we will discover in ourselves hitherto unknown abilities, our true vocations, our higher potentialities which seek to express themselves.

To paraphrase this in slightly more modern language: *attaining the goal of self-realisation begins with getting to know and mastering our personality. This involves an inner exploration of our lower, middle and higher unconscious, in other words, working on ourselves at different levels, to discover our true abilities and higher potentialities, and thus engaging self-actualisation. This leads to the recognition and realisation of our true or higher Self, which becomes the unifying centre for our further development – transpersonal psychosynthesis.*

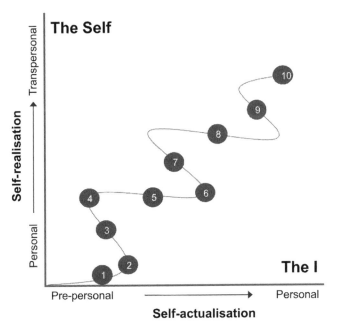

Figure 3.3 Example life journey along the two dimensions of self-development.

Within this, the starting point and main focus of the work of personal development is best summarised as *getting to know and mastering our personality, through exploring all levels of our consciousness*. This is an important message both to ourselves as coaches and for those we are coaching, and gets missed in more superficial approaches to personal development that only emphasise developing skills and behaviour.

Finally, let me use my own life as a (highly simplified) example of the interplay of these two dimensions – following every appearance of outward success at school (1), I hit a crisis of identity and meaning as a young adult at university (2), that led to an inner search for truth and understanding of who I was (3), in which I embarked upon a path that led to a series of peak experiences and profound self-realisation (4), liberating me to express myself fully and experience an extended period of career achievement (5), culminating in a gradual return to self-doubt and questioning at a deeper level (6), leading me to engage in a rich period of personal and professional development (7), fuelling a new phase of actualisation in the organisational world (8), before responding to a pull towards my current work with psychosynthesis coaching, bringing inner healing and resolution (9), which I am now channelling into my courses and writing (10). Elsewhere in this book, I will unpack this journey in a little more detail, colouring in my personal development in terms of aspirations, strengths, issues and edges during each of these phases, as well as considering how this translates into Assagioli's language of personal and transpersonal psychosynthesis. For now, I simply want to show an example of how these phases illustrate cycling between periods of working on self-realisation and self-actualisation (Figure 3.3).

Having established this contextual foundation for how we might approach personal development as psychosynthesis coaches, we now turn outwards to the call for psychosynthesis coaching in the leadership and organisational world. We return to the unfolding theme of personal and professional development in Chapters 7 and 10.

A coaching story: *Going live*

William was not just an essential member of the leadership team: without him the whole project would probably have gone off the rails. He not only had a brain the size of the planet, knowing more about the technology than everyone else put together, he had been with the project from the start and understood how their platform was a finely balanced mesh of internal and external sticking plasters that could easily become unstuck. He knew this and so did everyone else. The problem, at least as William saw it, was that he didn't get on with the CEO. The other problem, which William didn't see so easily, was that everyone found him difficult to work with, and he often left a trail of confusion in his wake. As the date for going live got nearer and the project became more intense, the pressure was mounting on William and this state of affairs was becoming increasingly difficult to manage. He often felt stressed and isolated.

The CEO knew the coach from his previous project and hoped he could help William find a better way of working with the rest of the team. William welcomed the offer of coaching because he had ambitions to make the transition from 'technology expert' to a senior leadership position. At their first meeting William talked a lot about his personal and professional goals, as well as the problems in the organisation and the challenges he felt he was facing. The coach suggested they work together on a 360-feedback exercise to help William understand more accurately what his strengths and weaknesses were and identify key areas to work on in his development.

The feedback was very clear – everyone liked William and knew he was essentially a good person, but found him really difficult to work with, partly because he delighted in communicating the complexity of the project but mostly because his keen mind was always looking for the faults and risks in what others were doing. He saw this as serving the whole, but it didn't feel like that to those on the receiving end of his critical gaze. Using the feedback, the coach helped William to form some goals, including developing his emotional and social intelligence. They agreed to meet every two weeks for three months.

The coach wondered much about the tensions and contradictions in William's personality and his often incongruous behaviour. The coach saw someone with a very big heart (and good will), but without the emotional or relational skills to express it effectively. Someone who had developed a very keen mind as a way of surviving and succeeding in the world and channelled his desire to contribute down this single track. Someone with masses of resolve, determination and skilful (sometimes strong) will to make things happen but lacking an awareness or connection with his own or others' inner world.

Most sessions would start with the coach listening to William's story of what had been happening, the technical problems, the deadline dramas, the relationship issues. Eventually the coach would challenge William to look towards a deeper place by asking 'So that's the outer world, what's been happening in your inner world?', 'where are you in all this?', and 'what are you feeling now about that?' The coach offered examples of what it sounds like to disclose your inner dialogue. William was discovering a new language and starting to find a way to connect his mind and his heart. Each session they would identify and agree something new that William might try in the way he communicated and related with the team.

During one session William realised that his critical voice was an echo of critical voices from his past, particularly his father's. He started to see that this wasn't really him, it was just a part of him. The way his critical mind solved complex and difficult problems was core to the value he brought to the project, but it wasn't his whole identity. There were other parts to him which he could draw out, including an empathetic part that could listen to others without judgement. A deeper sense of what it meant for him to be a leader was starting to emerge.

In a subsequent session, William discovered something very important – people didn't know what he knew or was thinking unless he told them. This may sound something rather simple for someone so bright to miss, but that is often the case with really clever people. 'But it's obvious', he would often say. Obvious to you but maybe not to them, the coach would reply. You need to explain things so that people understand, if you want to bring them with you.

In another session, William described an important breakthrough with Alison, his key direct report. 'We went out for a coffee around the corner and chatted for half an hour, stepping outside of our usual day-to-day business. We can now both talk about what we are thinking and feeling and what we need from each other. It has completely changed the way we work together and we've agreed to keep doing this once a week'.

Alongside the coaching, the CEO created a new reporting structure which gave William a more sympathetic line manager. There were still some crises to be navigated but everyone in the team started to feel William was being more human and much easier to work with. Eventually the project successfully went live and everyone involved was happy. When the time was right, William was able to hand over his various roles to the business-as-usual team and started out on a new path that eventually led to a senior leadership position in the parent company.

Chapter 4

The leadership challenge and the call to coaching

What is the nature of the leadership challenge in today's organisations and society? How does psychosynthesis speak to today's crisis of leadership? In what ways is Roberto Assagioli's writing and teaching relevant and applicable to what is happening today?

An existential crisis of leadership

I will begin by exploring the emergent and unfolding crisis of leadership, which I have previously characterised as *the leadership gap* (Howard, 2017a-1).

As we might all recognise from our different experiences and perspectives, the organisational world and society in general are constantly changing and evolving, sometimes imperceptibly or gradually and sometimes clearly and quickly. I am frequently amazed to observe the capacity of human beings to adapt to new circumstances, confront new challenges, take on new ways of looking at things that only yesterday seemed alien or irrelevant.

But when does change (or an absence of change) become a crisis? What is the nature of our current societal crisis? How might we characterise this?

If we briefly survey society today (admittedly, outside of our own direct experience and areas of expertise, we are overly dependent upon a less than perfect media for this) there are recognisable crises in almost every direction we look: environment, climate, finance, politics, economy, market capitalism, equality, global interconnectedness, mental health, education, community, family, work, technology, etc. These might be characterised in terms of: unsustainability of current trends; worsening intractable and apparently unresolvable problems; complexities and interdependencies beyond current comprehension; inability to bring about desired outcomes or anticipate unintended consequences; an incapacity to find or implement effective solutions. I would argue that the common thread running through many if not all of these is *leadership* – in terms of lack of leadership, failure of leadership, questioning of leadership. Therefore, the crisis I want to focus on is that of leadership, which I characterise as an existential crisis, and which can be viewed at both individual and collective levels.

What do we mean by an existential crisis? Roger Evans, drawing upon Victor Frankl, provides a definition in his overview of the existential crisis of leadership, in *5DL: Five Dimensions of Leadership* (2020):

> By this term, I mean a moment when an individual or group questions the very foundations of their lives: whether what they are doing or trying to do or accomplish has any meaning, purpose or value. These moments (crises) often represent critical (key) turning points in our lives, in adolescence, in mid-life when we ask deeply is there another level of meaning or purpose trying to emerge and enter our lives.

He goes on to explain how the resolution of the crisis requires engagement at a different level to that which created it, with an openness to *'explore the essence of what is happening and wonder about what is trying to emerge'*. For the leadership crisis, *'this means shifting context and asking what is the essence or the heart of leadership'* beyond the current conventional characterisation of leadership in terms of competencies and models.

In my response to this challenge of *unravelling the essence of the existential leadership crisis* and *shifting the context to a new level*, I am going to propose that we need to understand and work with three inter-related themes at individual and collective levels: Complexity, Being and Will.

Complexity

Complexity is at the heart of the leadership crisis and is the primary driver of the growing leadership gap between the response needed and the capability available in relation to a crisis. Let me illustrate this with reference to three different commentators:

Jean Houston (2013), in an online article:

> ...too many of the problems in societies today stem from leadership that is ill-prepared to deal with present complexity. ...[T]oo many leaders have been educated for a different time, a different world. Few are prepared for the task of dealing with the complexity and chaos of today when the usual formulas and stop-gap solutions of an earlier era will not help.

Adam Curtis' latest documentary film of our times, HyperNormalisation (2016), echoes this state of affairs and tells the story of:

> How we got to this strange time of great uncertainty and confusion where those who are supposed to be in power are paralysed and have no idea what to do.

Robb Smith (2016, np) expands upon this analysis of what is often now referred to as VUCA (Volatility, Uncertainty, Complexity, Ambiguity):

> ...a rapidly-changing world that is, in many ways, moving too fast for all of us really is scary, uncomfortable and unsettling. We're connected in ways we haven't yet mastered, we're learning at rates we can't yet process and we are subject to forces we can't hope to understand (even experts don't really understand the complex dynamical systems at the core of their disciplines). We're all in this messy, chaotic process together.

These illustrate the collective-level challenge of complexity. At the individual level, leaders face increasing complexity in their organisational environments as well as inner lives, sometimes combining with pressure and stress to the point of overwhelm, shutout or breakdown. Dealing with complexity is a prime imperative for all of us and involves developing new levels of awareness, capacities for understanding and strategies for action. Specifically, we need to develop our capacity for taking systemic perspectives and engaging with systems forces (e.g. DL4 in Evans' five dimensions of leadership (2020). I emphasise the need for a systemic perspective here because, without it, we are simply overwhelmed by content and detail, or worse, we deny and reduce complexity to fit our comfort zone of over-simplification, with potentially disastrous consequences.

To help bring this down to a grounded experience at the individual level of leadership, I pose to leaders these challenging questions about complexity:

- What are the complexities of your outer organisational world? For example multiple stakeholders and partnerships; rapidly changing markets; internal processes and projects; hidden politics, loyalties and motivations...
- What are some of the complexities of your inner world? For example: conflicting needs and motivations; creating synergy between your worlds of relationship, work and self-understanding; aligning career direction with inner purpose and meaning; dealing with stress and crises...
- How good are you at living with uncertainty and ambiguity? Can you stay with not knowing? How much do you need to be in control? How do you assert your need to be in control in complex or chaotic situations? Or do you withdraw or cut off?
- How developed is your systemic awareness? Can you stand back from the human systems you are deeply involved in? Do you work with or against the systems forces in your organisation?

It is important to realise that systemic intelligence isn't just about systemic thinking (as so importantly introduced to a wider audience in Senge's *Fifth*

Discipline (1990)). We need to include ourselves in the picture, to combine big-picture cognitive awareness with our subjective experience of being. This is about bringing the psychospiritual perspective together with systemic thinking in order to develop effective systemic practice. And so we connect to our second theme: that of *being*.

Being

Leadership concerns **being**. That is, it concerns the *being* of leadership, versus the *doing* of leadership; how to *be* a leader; creating the space for the human *being* in the workplace; *being* in right-relationship. This *being* dimension of leadership is also sometimes approached in terms of self-and-other-awareness, presence or charisma. A door has also been opened to bringing or allowing the *being* to be more present in organisations through the growing popularity and acceptance of mindfulness practices.

Successful leadership is as much about *who* you are and *how* you are as about *what* you do. Most leadership development focuses almost entirely on the doing aspect of leadership: the competencies, skills and behaviours; the strategies, tactics and execution. Although the importance of leadership *being* is increasingly acknowledged, very little practical support or development of this dimension is offered. In spite of this, many good leadership coaches might naturally and intuitively 'bring their being' to their coaching and 'nurture the being' of their clients. This is where leadership coaching can play an important role, and why we are evolving psychosynthesis coaching. Central to our approach is the model of trifocal vision, which I also describe as *coaching the Being* (see Chapter 8).

'Coaching the being' involves opening your heart to the Being or the Self of the other, as a continuing or periodic reflective practice. In coaching supervision, Roger Evans invites us to ask the question 'As you open our heart to this person, who do you see?' The choice to open the heart enables us to see beyond our mind and transcend any psychological diagnosis to reach psycho-spiritual holding, awareness or presence. The engagement between the coach and the leader coachee thus aligns with the ever-present unconscious connection at the level of being (between the two beings) and a transformative space opens up. Even if this *opening of the heart* goes only one way (coach to leader), the potential for transformation enters the space, thus evoking the Self for the leader and enabling the Will of the Self of the leader to start to become expressed.

We (both coaches and leaders) very rarely find this easy given the busy-ness and clutter of both our inner lives and outer organisational worlds. As we grow and develop, our inner lives can actually become more complex and the impact of our unexplored history and unconscious drives more important – hence the need to explore our different levels (pre-personal, personal and transpersonal) of consciousness and unconsciousness, and the psychological processes that work away in our psyche.

'Coaching the being' helps create the context for what Frederic Laloux refers to as the principles of *wholeness*, evolutionary *purpose* and *self-organisation* in evolutionary organisations, which are responses to the challenge of the emerging leadership crisis.

To help bring this down to the individual level of leadership, I pose these challenging questions to leaders about *leadership being:*

- What does it mean to bring your being, who you are most essentially, to your role as a leader? To what extent do you feel you do this?
- Which parts of yourself do you bring to leadership and which parts do not come so easily? Can you be vulnerable in your role as leader? Are you open to feedback? Can you ask for help? Are you humble or hubristic?
- How comfortable are you with finding time to deeply reflect in your day-to-day work? Are you addicted to busy-ness and activity? In what ways?
- How quick are you to fill spaces and pauses in conversations and meetings with colleagues? Do you allow surprises, unexpected ideas or insights to happen around you?

I would like to suggest that *coaching the being* can support leaders in their capacity to deal with complexity – that these two themes are inter-connected. The proposition here is that we (and the leaders we are coaching) need to expand our inner awareness and capacities in order to be able to meet the outer challenges we are facing in the world. Meeting these outer challenges requires the engagement of my third theme: Will.

Will

I am proposing that the existential leadership crisis is also a crisis of **Will**. This is probably the least recognised aspect of the crisis in public discourse (whether in generalist media or specialist leadership and organisational forums), or, in other words, the most unconsciously held. I suggest that one of the reasons for this, paradoxically, is the over-emphasis on doing over being in leadership, and the confusion between free will and strong will. Action, performance, results, *doing*, become valued in themselves and disconnected from transpersonal purpose, will and intention. Action (can you make it happen?) becomes an obsessional, *strong-will* drive to the detriment of reflection and sense-making. The wider context for this is the prevailing rationalistic-scientific-materialistic paradigm of modern western society, and the corresponding bias for rational-behavioural models and approaches in business and organisational theory that close down, ignore or suppress the sensory-somatic and feeling-emotional levels of human experience in the workplace. This in turn shuts down our experience of being, our capacity to connect with Self and therefore Will as the first expression of Self.

Alongside this, individual agency has gradually got lost in the shadow of all-encompassing wider organisational and societal systems. Notice the high regard in which successful entrepreneurs and business people – the likes of Richard Branson, Steve Jobs and Jeff Bezos – are held. These are the exceptions to the norm – remarkable individuals, who against the odds, have been able to find and express their free will (or perhaps strong will?) through their life's passion, business project or serial entrepreneurship. Equally, society tends to celebrate exceptional sports people, film and television actors, artists and entertainers, who have achieved unique success amongst a very large field of potential contenders. Now, with the cult of celebrity, achieving fame has become an end in itself.

Free will in large business (also public service or third sector) organisations is a rare commodity. Mostly it seems limited to a small group of senior executives and then, on closer inspection, we might find those individuals at the top feel as trapped within the system as those in the middle or the bottom of the organisational system (drawing upon Barry Oshry's basic model in *Seeing Systems* (2007). Often the organisational system is a continuing expression and embodiment of the available free will of the founder of the business or originators of the organisation, even long after they have moved on or passed over control. The initial creation of value becomes enshrined in a system that then becomes a barrier to new value generation as new expressions of creative free will.

However, the endurance of past creation is rapidly lessening as market conditions change. In *The Second Curve* (2015) Charles Handy reminds us that the average life of a business has reduced from 40 years to 14 years, as a symptom of the speeding up of change cycles and the consequent need to keep reinventing ourselves, individually and collectively. He shows how the 'sigmoid curve' provides a useful metaphor for thinking about initiating change in our lives (as well as in our businesses and society) at the point when everything appears to be still going well (i.e. on the up-curve of our past creativity), rather than waiting for evidence of decline before acting. He cites Apple's successive initiations of the iPod, iPhone, iPad and iWatch as the classic example of successful second-curve thinking in business and ponders whether this will continue without Steve Jobs at the helm. While not naming it explicitly, Handy is talking about Will and the ability to act and direct our lives or our organisations rather than live in reaction to events.

Ironically, many organisational leaders then desperately seek ways to re-activate creative free will within their organisations, either through efforts to connect with transpersonal will and collective engagement with the organisation's purpose, vision or mission, or by encouraging individual agency through the development of leaders. On both pathways, if systems forces are not adequately recognised and addressed, there is little chance for success. The general level of cynicism about vision workshops, culture change, employee empowerment or engagement programmes in most large organisations is high. If the source or cause of the disempowerment or disengagement of people in the organisation is not tackled first, well-intentioned leadership and people strategies may simply add to the tangle of systems forces.

Against this backdrop, it becomes clearer to see what we are contending with when, as psychosynthesis coaches, we work with individual leaders to help them find, activate and nurture their free will.

It is important to recognise that the systems dynamics and forces at play in organisations and society have always been present (and clearly were in Assagioli's day, as we will see). We can argue that the degree and intensity has increased, along with a corresponding sense of isolation and powerlessness, or worse, no sensation at all as people unconsciously play out their parts within the system.

At the societal level, through the toxic combination of increasing or growing (i) complexity as illustrated earlier (*we don't know how to solve our problems anymore*), (ii) individual isolation and alienation, with the breakdown of traditional societal structures of family, friendship and community, which become replaced by corporatism, consumerism and social media (*we don't know how to be with and relate to others anymore*), (iii) global interconnectedness (*we depend upon people we have no relationship with*) and (iv) selective visibility of what is going on elsewhere in the world (*we see suffering, injustice or threat and feel powerless*), often through distorting combinations of new internet and old media, most people's sense of free will has become increasingly forlorn, frustrated and distorted. Pankaj Mishra (2016), a Guardian columnist, points towards the dangers of this:

> ...we cannot understand this crisis because our dominant intellectual concepts and categories seem unable to process an explosion of uncontrolled forces... we find ourselves in an age of anger, with authoritarian leaders manipulating the cynicism and discontent of furious majorities.

In conclusion, I would argue that, to a large degree, we have reached a state of affairs where individual agency and free will appear to have become suppressed or subordinated within the bigger system – be that the corporate system of large organisations, or the western consumer society system or wider global systems.

I believe that this state of affairs is being unconsciously compounded by what is happening at the intellectual, academic or ideas level – with the advent of a new determinism in the form of neuroscience (or neuropsychology). There is much of enormous value that has come out of this rapidly emerging and quickly spreading field. At the very least it can be seen to provide scientific evidence for much of what humanistic, transpersonal or psychospiritual psychologists have been saying for years. But this might come at a price – the wolf of scientific materialism in human clothing, the potential for colonisation of the subjective realms of knowledge by this super new objective realm of knowledge. At the end of this colonisation, there might be little space left for the soul or the human spirit, or for free will, individual agency, ultimate values or universal Self. If you follow the collective thrust of neuropsychology, the unconscious becomes all powerful, wider systems and social forces all pervasive, our capacity for individual agency and free will delusional in the knowledge of our genetic makeup and animal nature, and Self or self an illusion because it cannot be located in the brain. In other words, we are left to confront a rather deterministic world. For this we need an antidote – which I suggest is rediscovery of the Will.

In this section I have been seeking to unravel the essence of the existential leadership crisis through exploring the relationship between the three themes of Complexity, Being and Will. Without directly drawing upon Assagioli's work, I have shown the need or calling for a psychospiritual psychology of Self and Will, in other words Assagioli's psychosynthesis, as part of the response to the existential crisis of leadership at a qualitatively different level.

Within this context, I want to turn again to Assagioli's key work, *The Act of Will* (1974), and look for new ways in which this wisdom from the past might help us with the current crisis, which I will do in Chapter 16.

Individual and collective levels

At the start I suggested we need to explore the leadership gap at both the individual and the collective levels.

At an **individual level**, leaders face increasing complexity in their organisational environments as well as their inner lives, sometimes combining with pressure and stress to the point of overwhelm, shutout, breakdown or crisis. Dealing with complexity is a prime imperative for all of us and involves developing new levels of awareness, capacities for understanding and strategies for action. Let me ask you to reflect upon the following questions:

1   In what ways does this resonate with your experience of working with the challenge of complexity? Or with the being of leadership? What would you add or say differently?
2   What are you learning about engaging with and closing the leadership gap in your own practice with leaders?
3   How do we see the leadership gap in relationship to leadership development? Is this about helping leaders shift or transform in their mix of action logics, worldviews or paradigms? Or more about responding to what is emergent in the leader? Or helping them develop a capacity of inner complexity that matches the outer complexity?

At the **collective level**, the gap between the leadership that is needed and the leadership capability that is available seems to be widening, with potentially serious consequences for both organisations and society.

1   How does this shape the agenda for leadership education, development and coaching?
2   How might we think differently about addressing this gap?
3   How might leadership development in organisations help, inform or cross over to leadership development in society (e.g. politicians, communities) more widely?

A coaching story: *Stepping up*

Katrina had recently joined the leadership team, appointed by Frank as the head of a new department, set up to revolutionise the way that the company developed new products. Initially everyone in the team was friendly and polite to her, if a little aloof and distant.

After the novelty and sense of intimidation wore off, she started to notice how complacent most of the team seemed about the big challenges the organisation was facing and how most interactions in the team were carefully guarded political manoeuvres undertaken by each leader to protect their territory. She started to challenge her colleagues on technical as well as strategic issues, which sometimes led to uncomfortable tensions in the group. She was invited to attend the annual Senior Leaders Conference for the whole organisation and did her best to engage in all the social gatherings, but always felt like an outsider at an exclusive 'boys club'. At her annual review, Frank gave her much positive feedback about her overall contribution and the dynamic team she had set up. However, he also wanted her to learn to be more diplomatic, more patient with the process of change and to create less conflict in the way she worked.

She brought this feedback to a session with her leadership coach and asked how she should respond. The coach asked her what she thought was going on here. Her first response was that *'Frank is very conflict averse and I make him feel uncomfortable. The members of his team are comfortably feathering their nests and avoid dealing with the real issues'.* Yes, all that's true. What else is going on? *'The system is entrenched in a very male-dominated world view and it's very difficult for a woman to be accepted as a leader unless one behaves like the boys'.* Yes, that's also true. And what else? *'I feel suddenly caught and triggered by people to react in ways I don't seem to have any choice about. I get upset, feel isolated and can't see a way out'.* Good; would you like to work on freeing yourself from these reactions and patterns?

Thus Katrina and the coach started to explore the thought patterns, feelings and behaviours associated with her experiences of being caught and trapped. They found a key limiting mindset which traced all the way back to her childhood and the family dynamic with her siblings. By following a process of awareness, recognition, integration and synthesis, Katrina started to build the place of acceptance and compassion for herself that had been missing in her early life. Alongside working with the past, they examined how old patterns reflected in the way she related with her colleagues today.

The coach wondered much about Katrina and the way that she was developing as a leader and who she was becoming. She had grown incredibly over the period they had been working together. She was much more resilient, confident, self-aware and socially competent than when they had met, and yet there were still shadows from the past that haunted her. Most of her life she had been driven by her need to prove herself and this had contributed to considerable academic achievement and a rapid rise in her professional and corporate career. She still struggled with her demons, although now much less so than in the past, and could recognise when aspects of her personality were caught by people and situations. Her latest promotion was a step change and called for a new way of being as well as acting as a leader.

She started to build alliances and friendships with members of her peer team and realised that some of them weren't so bad and actually saw things the same way as she did. Frank asked her to lead the strategic review for the organisation alongside her current role, and she initiated a series of cross-organisational workshops, supported by her coach and others. This led to what came to be seen as the organisation's most successful cultural and behavioural change project, which made a lasting difference to the way that people worked together.

Chapter 5

Coaching psychology

Why does coaching need to be underpinned by psychology? Why does leadership coaching need a psychospiritual psychology?

Why coaching needs psychology

It is now fairly widely accepted in the coaching world that good coaching needs to be underpinned by coaching psychology in some way, in terms of the education and training of coaches, their understanding of themselves and their clients, as well as the approaches and methods they bring to their practice. Beyond that, there is not much consensus about what that looks like, and there is much variety and experimentation in both theory and practice.

The application of psychology is one of the key ways by which coaching becomes differentiated from other forms of helping or working relationships, such as management, mentoring or consulting. Much early business coaching in the 1980s and 90s involved ex-leaders, managers and consultants offering one-to-one coaching on the basis of their business skills, experience and knowledge rather than specific coaching skills or psychological competence. Early efforts to professionalise coaching focused on identifying and developing the key skills of coaching, and much coach training still focuses on such skills development. This is reflected in the ICF competencies framework, summarised below (as listed in Whittaker, 2017):

- Meeting ethical guidelines and professional standards
- Establishing the coaching agreement
- Establishing trust and intimacy with the client
- Coaching presence
- Active listening
- Powerful questioning
- Direct communication
- Creating awareness
- Designing actions

- Planning and goal-setting
- Managing progress and accountability

Against this backdrop, in 1992, Sir John Whitmore wrote in the first edition of his seminal *Performance for Coaching (p16)*:

> In too many cases they (coaches) have not fully understood the performance-related psychological principles on which coaching is based. Without this understanding they may go through the motions of coaching or use the behaviours associated with coaching, such as questioning, but fail to achieve the intended results.

Much has changed since 1992, not least that client expectations and competition amongst coaches have increased, at the same time as different psychologies have found ways to make themselves relevant and applicable in the organisational world. Alongside this, there has been a gradual migration of practitioners from counselling and therapy into coaching, bringing their psychological training and approaches with them. Julia Bueno summarises the fusion fuelling the rise of coaching (2010):

> One view is that coaching reflects a synthesis of three movements: the growth of the talking therapies; consulting and organisational development and industrial psychology; and the proliferation of personal development trainings.

The growth of personal development has been a significant influence, leading organisational clients to become more familiar themselves with various forms of psychology and therefore more likely to expect and be ready to embrace psychological engagement from the coaches with whom they work.

We must now pause and recognise that psychology is a very broad field. As far as coaching is concerned, most psychology leans towards the behavioural and is focused on the outer, observable, measurable world of the client – performance improvement, behavioural change and skills development – rather than their inner world or on personal development at a deeper level. This has coincided with a more general trend in organisational development to focus very intensely on behaviour and performance improvement.

A recent survey of 2,791 coaches as part of a 2017 report on *The State of Play in European Coaching and Mentoring* asked which approaches coaches used in their practice (see Figure 5.1).

The survey also asked which approaches coaches had been trained in, with a level of responses very similar to the question about usage in their practice. A curious anomaly was that more coaches used *motivational interviewing* than are trained in this approach, which suggests coaches ticked this option either not really knowing what it means or having only read something about it.

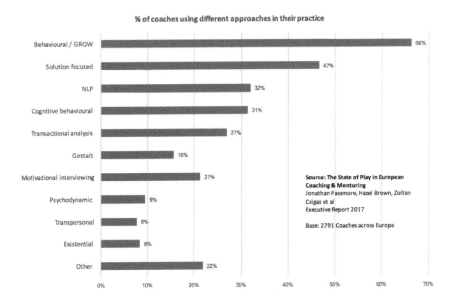

% of coaches using different approaches in their practice

Figure 5.1 Approaches used by coaches in their practice.

(Source: Passmore, Jonathan; Brown, Hazel; Csigas, Zoltan et al. (2017), *The State of Play in European Coaching & Mentoring*, Executive Report 2017)

Overall, the figures suggest that most coaches use the GROW model and draw upon two or three other approaches. It is not clear whether training in these is in-depth (e.g. Masters/postgraduate level) or consists of short courses (self-certification etc.) or basic introductions.

I would argue that it is not enough to simply have (i) an understanding of the psychological principles underlying coaching as described by Whitmore and (ii) to apply one or more of the psychological approaches listed above, but that (iii) coaching also needs to be underpinned by what I call a core coaching psychology, which provides the coach with grounded psychological depth and even a guiding philosophy to their approach. Most of the above-mentioned psychologies are used as core coaching psychologies by some coaches, although I would suggest some are better suited to this purpose than others. Gestalt psychology offers itself as a core coaching psychology (see Peter Bluckert, 2006) and many practitioners draw upon Transactional Analysis in a similar way. The integrative approach which draws upon elements of psychodynamic, humanistic and transpersonal psychology is also popular (e.g. in courses run by Metanoia) and is probably the closest to psychosynthesis in providing a model of Self/self. However, Gestalt and TA, Neurolinguistic Programming (NLP) and many other popular coaching psychologies lack a central model of the Self and this is a serious impediment to working at the level of the being. It will become clearer why this is important as we more fully unpack psychosynthesis as a coaching psychology in the next chapter.

Why leadership coaching needs a psychospiritual psychology

Put simply, there is an emerging and growing crisis of leadership that I suggest calls out for a psycho-spiritual perspective. I recently touched upon the nature of this crisis in a blog post on *the leadership gap* (Howard, 2017a). The crisis of leadership can generally be explored at three levels: individual, organisational and societal. The societal crisis of leadership, in particular in politics both nationally and globally, continues to be widely observed and commented on in our media and beyond. This whole topic, and how a psycho-spiritual approach can help, deserves a fuller treatment than I can give here, so below I focus on what it means at the individual and organisational levels for coaches.

Individual leadership crisis

The organisational and leadership landscape has changed significantly since coaching first started to become accepted and even commonplace in our organisations. As we all know and are frequently reminded, organisations are being increasingly impacted by change, uncertainty and complexity, and need to become more innovative, collaborative and adaptive. What isn't talked about so much is how the fundamental relationship between the individual and the organisation is changing and what this means for both leaders and coaches. The typical individual leader is facing mounting organisational challenges and performance pressures that bring corresponding personal stress and psychological pressures. Being a leader these days has a very personal dimension that needs to be recognised and supported.

The personal has become very much part of the territory – partly in a positive and overt way, for example in organisations wanting people to bring their whole selves to work: their energy, resourcefulness, ambitions, passions and purposes. It is also partly in a less positive or shadow way, for example as with leaders who are working under enormous pressure to produce results to the point of generating unhealthy levels of stress, or experiencing very personal inner crises (e.g. of identity and meaning – who am I and why am I here?) that are intricately connected with their role as leader. Issues of work–life balance can confront people at every level of an organisation, as can ethical conflicts that are not openly talked about. Boundaries (e.g. what is business-personal and what is personal-private?) are fuzzy, shifting and becoming increasingly multi-dimensional and complex. Coaches therefore need to be able to work with personal and psychological dimensions alongside the business and practical.

It is also important to include the broader impact of leadership and management development over recent years. The prevailing individualistic, economic and career-oriented nature of the dominant MBA culture has not equipped senior leaders well to meet the kinds of crisis in which they may find themselves. Starkey and Hall set out to challenge the prevailing MBA narrative in *The Spirit of Leadership* (2012, p82), in which:

> we explain how we aim to develop an alternative management and leadership narrative from a mind-set that emphasizes humanity, plurality, and reflexivity. To do this, we aim in our teaching to promote an authentic learning community defined by critical self-reflection and intercultural learning to challenge the lure of a narcissistic, self-preoccupied individualism that often goes with power and wealth.

Roger Evans in *Five Dimensions of Leadership* (2020) goes further, to describe a growing existential crisis in which leaders must:

> realise that they are not only part of a whole, that they do not and cannot know everything, and that they must not try to do it all themselves. This demands significant insight and reflexivity. It goes straight to the heart of the crises of leadership that always happen when leaders think they know all the answers and that there are no alternatives to their heroic visions.

What does this mean for coaching? First of all, that leaders need help and support and that their openness to working with a coach is a very significant first step. However, most coaching has been focused on performance improvement, modifying behaviours or managing change, with a secondary focus on personal development that may support the leader to achieve their objectives in these areas. To the extent that psychology or psychological approaches have become part of the coach's context, method or toolkit, the emphasis has been on behaviourally oriented psychologies, such as CBT and NLP, or the newer positive- or neuro-psychologies that can also be highly effective at supporting performance improvement.

There is a place for all of this, and performance improvement is not a bad starting point for a coach in their practice, particularly when working with achievement-centred leaders (see Chapter 13). At the same time, many leaders now need a more balanced approach, which places equal emphasis on the inner and outer dimensions of their lives as leaders. Such an approach can support them in dealing with the business and the personal, with the light and the dark, with depth and height, with higher purpose and meaning, as well as with day-to-day challenges and sometimes the shadows. Some coaching focuses exclusively on the positive and ignores these shadows, the parts of ourselves and our consciousness we are less ready to acknowledge, such as echoes of trauma, suffering and our history, or how we have learned to survive as a personality. I am not suggesting the coach should work on healing the past, but these aspects can be very present and relevant to the coaching conversation and as such may need to be recognised, acknowledged and included.

Organisational leadership crisis

The developmental psychology perspective provides a map of how individuals, teams and organisations evolve and develop over time, as described in terms of organisational paradigms and leadership styles (Laloux, 2014). In a nutshell, Laloux describes seven organisational paradigms that broadly follow the emergence of human consciousness and societal worldviews over thousands of years of human history, and mirror the developmental stages that individuals work through as they grow up and mature in adulthood (at least in potentiality). These paradigms are the Reactive, Magic, Impulsive, Conformist, Achievement, Pluralistic and Evolutionary. It may help to think of these as ways of thinking and operating in the world, which are more or less activated within an individual, group, organisation or society depending upon history, circumstance and situational factors. With his book *Reinventing Organisations* Laloux explores examples of the emerging Evolutionary paradigm and examines the three common principles of self-organisation, wholeness and evolutionary purpose that he finds help to activate this paradigm.

One simple way of characterising the current leadership crisis in organisations (and there are many) is that the current challenges and crises organisations are facing (e.g. complexity, agility, purpose, engagement etc.) require an Evolutionary response, but are largely met with leadership centred in the Achievement or Pluralistic paradigms. Laloux focuses on organisational development towards the Evolutionary paradigm, whereas it is often more relevant and practical to think about how to develop pockets of Evolutionary leadership (e.g. in key roles) within largely Achievement–Pluralistic organisations.

If you are working with a leader who is awakening to the Evolutionary paradigm, you will benefit from the context and methodology of a psychospiritual psychology, both when working with issues of wholeness and evolutionary purpose and when helping leaders in their vertical development. Often such leaders experience a crisis of transition, whether that be a crisis of meaning or duality or some form of spiritual awakening. Training in a psychospiritual psychology is important both for recognising what is happening for the client and knowing how to support them. More generally, there is a growing need to include and address the whole human being in organisations – so we need a psychology that includes the whole human being to help us do this.

Psychosynthesis provides the psychospiritual context, methods and tools to help us to explore working at this level. Although I know from my own experience that any experiential group can activate learning at this level of being, it also helps to have the structure and grammar of a psychospiritual psychology to explore it more deeply. This is where we now go in the next chapter.

Chapter 6

Psychosynthesis as a coaching psychology

What does psychosynthesis provide as a core coaching psychology? How do key concepts of psychosynthesis, including the Will and Self, inform, guide and support leadership coaching?

What is psychospiritual psychology?

Psychosynthesis is a psychospiritual psychology of Self and Will that was developed by Roberto Assagioli. Quite a mouthful – so what does that mean? First of all, it is concerned with the whole human being-with the human psyche and all levels of our consciousness and unconsciousness. Explicitly this includes (i) the **higher** unconscious or superconscious, otherwise described as the transpersonal or spiritual realm; (ii) the **middle** unconscious, or realm of our personality and personal psychology; (iii) the **lower** unconscious, the realm of history, trauma and pre-personal psychology.

We sometimes describe psychosynthesis as a *holistic* psychology for including all these levels (whereas, say, psychoanalysis focuses only on the lower level); at other times we call it *integrative* for its capacity to bring together different psychologies into a relational whole. *Psycho-spiritual*, however, says it most distinctively, because it emphasises the relationship and interplay between the psyche (lower, middle and higher consciousness) and the spiritual, transpersonal or higher Self. Psychosynthesis (see Assagioli's egg diagram below) offers an explicit model of the human psyche that includes the Self. Psychologies that have no such central model of self often lack coherence (viz. NLP, Gestalt or TA – I say this having worked with all three of these modalities). It is important for coaches (and therapists for that matter) to have a model or concept of the psyche that includes the Self, because without one, we can lose sight of the being and get caught in the processes and contents of the mind.

Transpersonal and *psychospiritual* psychology are often conflated, but there is an important distinction between them. The former focuses on working

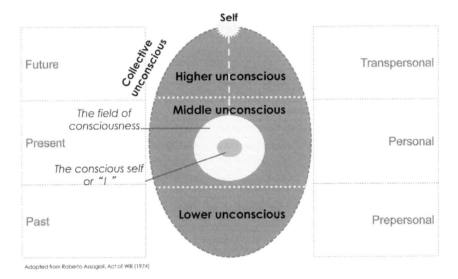

Adapted from Roberto Assagioli, Act of Will (1974)

Figure 6.1 Structure of the psyche – Roberto Assagioli.
Adapted for PGCPLC coach training programme.

at the transpersonal level, the latter with all levels. I would like to stress, as Assagioli does, the validity of a basic principle of psychosynthesis, which is that we can benefit from and use every function and element of our psyche (lower, middle and higher unconscious), provided we understand its nature and purpose and place it in its right relation with the greater whole (see Figure 6.1).

[A quick aside about the use of the word spiritual – we are using it here in the phenomenological sense to describe higher aspects of subjectively experienced consciousness. We are not concerned with religion or even spiritual practice and psychosynthesis as such is neutral with respect to these. It is also neutral in relation to new-age or alternative conceptions of spirituality that tend to be over-associated with what is called the pluralistic or relativistic paradigm.]

What do we mean by Self (with a capital S)? Assagioli explains (in *The Superconscious and the Self*, 1974, p1):

The transpersonal Self is basically ontological. Onthos means being – which is not process, but is something standing in itself. Self is the unchanging, enduring reality; a stable centre of life on its own level, which has functions but is not a function.

Perhaps a more familiar way of talking about this is in terms of our *being* – who we are most essentially; how we experience ourselves when we are most present. This is a question we encourage psychosynthesis coaches to reflect upon when working with someone – who is this being most essentially? If I open my heart to them, who do I see? What is emergent? Thus, we start with the Self, who this person or being is most essentially, and we remind ourselves that we are *coaching the being*, before the doing or the behaviour.

How are we coaching the being? We work with Self and Will and how these are experienced and manifest in the world, for example towards self-realisation and self-actualisation. Of course, any coaching also involves working with action and behaviour but the context for psychosynthesis coaching is to first hold awareness of and to reflect upon the *being*.

Psychosynthesis is also a psychology of Will, again using capital W to indicate our Transpersonal Will as distinct from our everyday strong will, skilful will and goodwill, which are aspects of will. We often say that Will is the first expression of Self; it is the way in which *who we are* comes into the world, the essential act of will that also manifests with our conscious experience of I or everyday self. Will is therefore next to Self and comes before the various psychological functions of the mind. Healthy and well-rounded will has the capacity to focus and direct the psychological functions of our minds – thinking, feeling, sensation, intuition, imagination, desire, etc., in service of Self (see Figure 6.2). However, much of the time we experience the reverse, with our will blocked or distorted by aspects of our personality and the way that our minds work.

Will is not the same as motivation – motivations can come from any part of our personality or mind and don't necessarily spring from our will to realise or actualise ourselves in the world. So a major difference between psychosynthesis coaching and more behavioural approaches is that we are seeking to help the client release or activate their will in relationship to their purpose and goals, rather than helping them find their motivation for doing things (although this may be a consequence of activating will).

How is this essentially different from conventional psychology?

Psychospiritual psychology challenges and changes the basic orientation of conventional psychology from **human *doing*** – so looking at the mind and how it dictates and influences our behaviour (British Psychological Society definition); in other words, *how* humans work and *what* they do – towards **human *being***: *who* we are most essentially; *how* we function as human beings; and within *that*, how the mind works and influences our behaviour. This shift re-orientates the direction of psychological inquiry into a new sequence, from **who** we are (Self/Being), to **why** we are (Will), to **how** we work (mind/body) and **what** we do (action/behaviour). This is the converse of the conventional sequence from *what* we do (behaviour), to *why* we do it (motivation), to *how*

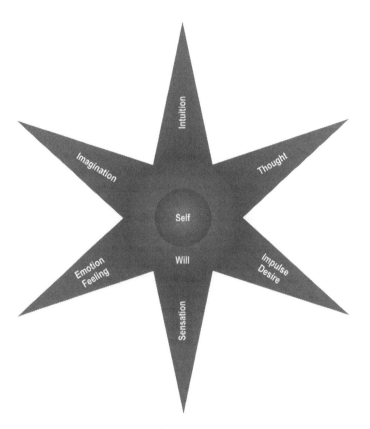

Figure 6.2 Assagioli's psychological functions.
From Assagioli, *The Act of Will* (1974).

that works (mind), and then to *who* is doing it. It may be easier to follow this in Figure 6.3 below.

With the conventional sequence, the Self is lost or never found. Neuroscientists cannot find a place in the brain where the Self/self/I exists and end up concluding that it is an illusion or a figment of our imagination created by our ego functioning. The evidence of our subjective experience of consciousness and the value of inner inquiry is discounted or ignored and we end up in a world where the Self no longer exists. This can have consequences for us all, not just individually but in society as a whole.

The original meaning of the word psychology (from the Greek – *psyche* and *logos*) was the *study of the soul*. I suggest modern psychology has somewhat lost its way through successive attempts to become more scientific, which ironically have led only to it becoming more partial and, philosophically at

Psychospiritual psychology

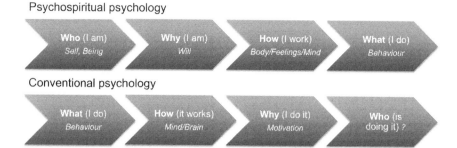

Figure 6.3 Two pathways of inquiry for psychology.

least, less scientific (see Wilber's *A Theory of Everything* (2000) if you are new to this argument and want to explore it). Ramesh Bijlani (2014, np) tells a succinct version of the story of how this happened:

> Psychology, in order to assert its status as a science, underwent a voluntary amputation. It got rid of those elements which did not fit within the framework of science. The first thing that it got rid of was the soul, because science denied the Divine, of which soul is the essence. Consequently, psychology became the study of the mind. However, even the mind is difficult to quantify. Hence psychology gradually became the study of behaviour.

Neal Goldsmith, in a post on Psychology Today (2010), seeks to '*bring psychologists, my clients, and us all back to psychology as the study of the psyche, to a focus on the ground of our being, to the soul, because it is this part of us that is the earliest, deepest, and the most authentic part of us*'.

Psychology has deep roots and perhaps it can find a way back to include the soul or Self again. We can also go back to draw upon shamanic wisdom, which looks at the four points of the medicine wheel and invites us to ask the questions 'Who am I? Why am I here? Where have I come from? And Where am I going?' – although not quite the same as my questions, these follow a similar direction of inquiry.

How do we apply psychology to leadership coaching?

What do we *mean* when we talk about applying – or bringing or drawing upon – any psychology in relationship to coaching? We actually mean some quite different things that are usually not well distinguished and can lead to confusion and even poor practice.

I have found that it helps to distinguish three different spaces in which we can apply a psychospiritual psychology as a coach. These are the *coach's* space, the *client's* space and the *coaching* space.

The coach's space

First, we should attend to how any psychology we are studying applies to us and **our personal and professional development**. This is particularly true for psychospiritual psychology, where our subjective knowledge and experience of the territory is so valuable when it comes to supporting clients. All self-aware professional practitioners already know the work always starts with themselves, that inner development informs outer inquiry and practice. In hindsight, this is how I first drew upon psychosynthesis for many years before I started using more explicit models of psycho-spiritual coaching (such as trifocal vision).

A mature, experienced and highly competent student on one of our coaching courses recently shared that, for her, personal development never ceases and that her experience of effectiveness and mastery as a coach has directly increased in proportion to her work on herself. My experience is the same. From this perspective as coaches we work on ourselves to increase our capacity to be with and know ourselves, which transfers directly to our capacity to be with and support our clients – what an amazing profession to be in! Contrast this with conventional academic psychology that seems to miss the practitioner entirely except as a thinking machine that observes, analyses and diagnoses what is going on 'over there'.

The client's space

Second, we can consider how psychology can be used directly in working with or on the **client's personal process or development;** for example using a specific technique, exercise or method, either formally or informally, working at the pre-personal, personal and transpersonal levels described earlier. For example this might include using guided visualisation to catalyse transpersonal creative expression, mindset reframing for addressing personal-level blocks to change, and identifying and owning projections in difficult relationships as a simple pre-personal-level intervention.

Working at the pre-personal level is where the greatest caution is needed, and there are boundary issues between coaching and therapy or counselling that need to be recognised (see Chapter 9 on therapy and coaching) – for example as coaches we do not engage directly in the therapeutic process with our client, although we may contextualise it, refer to it and even support action towards it.

Many practitioners rush too quickly and eagerly to use their chosen psychology to work on the client and I tend to caution against this: don't bring a technique to coaching for the sake of it; do so only in response to an emergent need or working in the gap to address blocks or impasses. The most common example I have come across is the zealous NLP practitioner using technique after technique with a client, intoxicated by the magic of instant apparent change. With some clients, I may never formally introduce a technique because all the important work happens naturally and informally in the coaching space.

The coaching space

So, thirdly and perhaps most importantly, our understanding of psychology can consciously and unconsciously inform and influence the **coaching space**, the coach's engagement with the coachee in the coaching session – the coaching conversation, dialogue, process or journey – however you want to characterise it. This alchemical space naturally touches upon and weaves between all levels of consciousness, all dimensions of time and the inner and outer lives of our clients as we follow the coaching process in service of the client's goals, purpose or needs.

As psycho-spiritual coaches, we hold awareness of the Self of the other as we explore the current reality and work in the gap to release available free will (trifocal vision). This creates a right-relational being space, which is where the mystery can be present and magic can happen, mixed up with more prosaic progress towards good outcomes from hard work, usually involving helping the client identify and take the next small step towards their goal. You may recognise this transformative space (sometimes experienced as a state of grace) that can enter the coaching space in the way that you work – it obviously doesn't need you to have studied psychospiritual psychology, but I recommend doing so if you want to develop your understanding of and capacity for recreating the transformative space.

Much more can be said about working in this transformative space as a coach and how it differs from working on the client's process. For a start, we bring our authentic presence as a coach; we can use ourselves as an instrument of change; we can bring ourselves as a resource – but always within the context of the coaching process and in service to the client's Self and Will, or – as Sir John Whitmore contextualises – for increasing the client's awareness and responsibility.

The three spaces are summarised in the graphic below which shows that, in effect, we are working at three levels in three spaces (see Figure 6.4) – so there are nine dimensions in all for applying psychospiritual psychology!

Why is this important? For new or inexperienced coaches, it helps to break down the task at hand for bringing psychology to their learning and practice, to gain perspective and prioritise their own learning. For more experienced coaches, this model helps us identify where we are strong and perhaps where we are weak or blind. It helps us navigate the territory of coaching and increases our options.

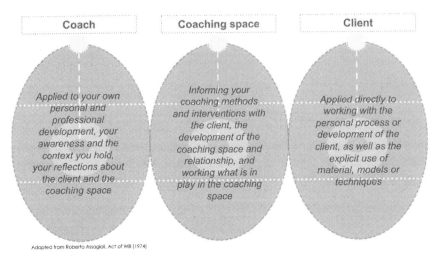

Coach

Applied to your own personal and professional development, your awareness and the context you hold, your reflections about the client and the coaching space

Coaching space

Informing your coaching methods and interventions with the client, the development of the coaching space and relationship, and working what is in play in the coaching space

Client

Applied directly to working with the personal process or development of the client, as well as the explicit use of material, models or techniques

Adapted from Roberto Assagioli, Act of Will (1974)

Figure 6.4 Three spaces for applying psychospiritual psychology in coaching.

Orientation and domain	Inner world and agendas/ *Being*	Outer world and agendas/ *Doing*
Past	Healing *Trauma, reflection, understanding*	Resolution *Sense making, acceptance, completion*
Present	Inner crisis and change *Self, personality, awareness*	Outer crisis and change *Systems, relationships, solutions*
Near future	Personal development *Will, capacity, growth*	Performance development *Behaviours, skills, action*
Far future	Self-realisation *Purpose, meaning, values*	Self-actualisation *Potential, career, leadership*

Goal or outcome focus
Outer and inner Reality
Options opportunities and resources
Activating Will and taking action

Context, Contract, Client, Capability

Figure 6.5 The territory of coaching.

Figure 6.5 below describes similar territory, but from the perspective of leadership coaching agendas, process and context.

To be capable and comfortable working across this broad territory the leadership coach can benefit from being grounded in a psycho-spiritual approach. This allows them to work with leaders in two domains: the *inner* domain, of personality and self, raising awareness of mindsets, attitudes and emotions and with the higher realms of purpose, meaning, values and identity; and the *outer* domain of behaviour and change. Coaches need to draw from a psychology that is concerned with the whole human being – essentially, we are describing a psychospiritual psychology such as psychosynthesis.

It is important to say that many experienced coaches working successfully in this way with *being* and *doing* (and I have met many who are members of APECS) have arrived at their current state of personal and professional development through their own unique learning journey, in which they have brought together different eclectic experiences (e.g. as leaders as well as coaches), approaches (e.g. leadership, Organisational Development and coaching models) or disciplines (e.g. backgrounds in psychology, counselling or therapy) – in effect they have internally created their own holistic or integrative approach. Psychosynthesis simply offers a more direct path to internalising a psychospiritual psychology for those setting out on this journey or those wishing to go further.

Dimensions, levels or elements at play within the leadership coaching space include:

- Levels of engagement – *what level are you working at as a coach? Who is your client?*

  - Individual – team – system

- Coaching agendas – *which agendas is your client bringing, both explicitly and implicitly?*

  - Inner: change, development, purpose; personal, being, self-reflection, inquiry
  - Outer: change, behaviour, performance; practical, planning, action, review

- Coaching horizon – *when in time is the client's energy blocked or needs attention? What is their temporal orientation?*

  - Past – present – future (near to far)

- Levels of consciousness – *which levels of consciousness are engaged? Where are the unconscious blocks?*

  - Pre-personal – personal – transpersonal

- Body – feelings – mind – *what parts of their experience does the client access easily? Which aspects are suppressed?*

  - Somatic awareness – emotional intelligence – mindsets and thought patterns

- Leadership development – *what are the priorities for the client's development? For example skills, intelligences, worldviews, self-esteem, confidence, awareness, will? What are the key interdependencies?*

- Horizontal – vertical – inner
- Focus on awareness and will – see *Five Dimensions of Leadership, Evans* (2020): for example self-awareness, awareness of others, systemic awareness, availability of free will, humility and openness to help

As psychosynthesis coaches we might touch upon any of these elements as we engage in the coaching process and support the awareness and responsibility of the client. We open up a transformative space, between the client's inner and outer worlds, where we are working with Self and Will across different domains according to the client's purpose, needs and goals. The coaching space thus becomes the crucible within which the mystery can enter and the alchemical process takes place. As the alchemist, the coach needs to hold this all very lightly or our rational mind may crush the crucible.

Chapter 7

Personal and professional
Part 2

> *The greatest revolution of our generation is the discovery that human beings,*
> *by changing the inner attitudes of their minds, can change the outer aspects*
> *of their lives.*
>
> William James, 1890

Part 2: seven perspectives on personal development for coaches

In Chapter 3 I described personal development as a vast and complex topic that can be approached in many different ways, interwoven as it is with the whole field of psychology, the story of the human potential movement, the leadership and talent development world, the popular self-help industry and of course the modern coaching profession. In the second part of this in-depth journey into personal development, I will explore various perspectives for coaches as a way of helping gain insight into this topic, whilst continuing the theme that personal development is a context to hold simultaneously for both ourselves and our clients.

It starts with an attitude

Personal development is about an attitude, an orientation, a choice and a commitment to yourself and the *idea* of personal growth. In what appears to be an increasingly deterministic world (at least according to the neuroscientists), your attitude is one thing you have choice and freedom about in your life. We always have the choice to nurture an attitude that embraces curiosity, openness to learning and some humility. Without these we easily start to crystallise and become fixed in our view, shape and pattern in the world. Indeed, our capacity to contain ambiguity, uncertainty and not-knowing – alongside continuing to inquire, discover and explore both the inner and outer world – shapes not just our path of personal development but also our ability to survive and adapt within an increasingly complex world.

There is a paradox at the heart of personal development, which is that however much progress we make we are also always starting out from where we are now. Although we might have worked on and developed ourselves over many years, it is our openness to continuing to develop and grow which makes the most difference to how we are as a coach. So, we are continuously facing the choice to renew our attitude, re-choose the path we have chosen. Even the best attitudes can become tired and stale and morph unconsciously into something less helpful. Attitudes are closely connected with moods and emotions, which can be coloured and changed by any little event of the day as well as over a longer period by all manner of situations in our lives. Therefore our attitudes need continuous, or at least periodic, reflection and renewal.

From this perspective, personal development can be a continuous process throughout our lives. To quote Roberto Assagioli, when asked whether there was a point of arrival or stable state at the end of the self-realisation journey:

> Life is movement, and the superconscious realms are in continuous renewal. In this adventure we move from revelation to revelation, from joy to joy. I hope you do not reach any 'stable state'. A 'stable state' is death.

Know thyself, know thy client

Personal development starts with self-awareness and the capacity to self-reflect. This then extends outwards to include our awareness of others, how they are different and how we impact upon and relate with them. Awareness and self-reflection are the starting point to knowing what 'our stuff" is and what our personality edges and developmental issues might be.

Essentially, we need to seek to know ourselves in order to know and work with others on their inner lives, to better understand and appreciate the psychospiritual territory in which we are working. Inner work with others is best accessed through our direct experience of our inner work on ourselves, rather than through the study and learning of theories and models (which then help in your own sense-making).

Within the psychosynthesis context, the coach is playing the role of a guide to the coachee in terms of their long-term psychospiritual development. We are using the term *guide* in a loose sense, in that it doesn't necessarily mean that the coachee is following the same developmental path as the coach (they may be very different to you), or even that the coach is ahead of the coachee on the path (as a therapist might regard themselves). Some coaches like to think of themselves as accompanying the coachee on their unique path, walking alongside them so to speak, and this can be a useful metaphor. What is important is that the coach has a living experience of what it means to be on their own psychospiritual developmental journey and is able, therefore, to guide and support the coachee in relationship to embarking on or continuing upon their own journey. There is also potential for synergy and a degree of reciprocity here, although not explicit – with the coach's personal development benefiting vicariously from the work the coachee is doing. At the same time, we must be wary of becoming too identified or self-referencing with our clients and remember that what was right for us may not be right for them.

> The more I understand myself, my identity, my business and direction and wider possibilities… the more this flows into my work with clients in helping them understand themselves, what they are doing and their direction… AY (PGCPLC student)

What's my stuff, what's their stuff?

We need to know our stuff so that we can be aware of when it is triggered and distinguish it from our client's stuff. If we are caught by our stuff when coaching and we are not aware of it or unconsciously react out of it, then we are not in the best place to serve our client. We need to be continuously curious, to ask ourselves as coaches in relationship to the other, what's my stuff and what's your stuff and how does my stuff get along with your stuff (e.g. do they play nicely together or get into a fight?).

What do I mean by 'stuff'? This term encapsulates our personality edges and issues, our blind spots and trigger-points, our unwanted patterns and preoccupations, wherever we have an emotional charge as a legacy from the past which can be activated automatically or unconsciously in different situations or by different types of people. *Where are you caught? Where do you get stuck? What reactivates you? What gets you into trouble in situations or relationships? What is my part in these problems that I experience?* These are the sort of questions that can help us inquire into our stuff and our baggage from the past. It is important to say that we should not be seeking to get rid of our stuff – rather to become more aware of it, to see when it is triggered and self-reflect at this point, to be able to own it and have a greater choice of response in relation to it. Over time, we might then notice that something (e.g. my anxiety when speaking in a large group, feeling intimidated by tall people, etc.) is no longer such an issue for me and that the focus for my development takes a new direction.

The psychological concepts that help us understand 'our stuff' include *transference and counter-transference*, as well as *projection and introjection*. Sometimes our client's stuff is reactivated simply by entering the situation of being coached, and can then be further triggered if we remind the client of someone from their past. We call this *transference*, and the way that you as the coach pick up that this is happening (usually in your emotional subconscious) we call *countertransference*. Transference can be positive (e.g. the coachee sees a good parental figure in the coach) or negative (the coach reminds the coachee of a harsh or critical parental figure). For the most part, the key thing for the coach is simply to be aware that this is going on and not to react to it, but to hold and contain the coachee and whatever might be going on for them. These concepts, how they tend to operate in coaching and how we might work with them, are an important focus on our coaching courses. For now, I am challenging you as the coach to consider situations or relationships where transference might be present for you (a clue: most authority figures – for example parent, boss, trainer, coach, therapist, supervisor, etc. – tend to activate some transference).

Ways of working on yourself

There are some subtleties to the meaning of the phrase 'working on yourself'. On one hand, I might say I am always working on myself within the context of personal development, at least in an ad-hoc informal way through ongoing reflection and deepening awareness (and sometimes I am really not working on myself, I am taking a break, hanging out, 'avoiding', not thinking too deeply, etc.).

On the other hand, there are specific actions, practices and activities we can engage in to work on ourselves, many of which might combine personal and professional development. The most obvious are personal and professional development courses and programmes, ranging from weekend seminars and retreats to Masters' degree-level programmes. Also included here is an engagement in any kind of helping professional relationship, whether coaching, counselling or psychotherapy, both individually and in group settings, both short- and longer-term. Then we have self-directed and individual practices, including any form of meditation, contemplation or mindfulness as perhaps the most commonly followed or prescribed. Obviously any self-study involving reading, reflecting and writing can be contextualised as a personal development practice, as might any mindful artistic and creative activity and certain physical practices or exercise routines such as yoga, qi gong, tai-chi or Pilates.

Self-reflection is obviously an important part of any personal development approach and can take many forms or be assisted by a variety of activities, coaching being an obvious one. Journal writing is a very common means of self-reflection and integration, for example in the form of an evening review, where you take time to reflect back upon the day: for example where did you get caught; what worked and what didn't. Attending retreats or spending extended time in contemplation or meditation is increasingly popular these days. Retreats can mean different things to different people and the distinction between personal development and spiritual practice can become blurred, although I don't see this as problematic – an activity can be contextualised in whatever way is most useful to the individual. For example for the last 10 years I have spent about an hour most days walking in nature as a way of reflecting upon and integrating what is happening in my life. At the same time, I consider this way of communing with nature as a spiritual practice, often finding myself in what I would describe as transpersonal states of consciousness. These are all just examples and ideas for personal development activities and practices, but really the options are endless and nothing should be excluded.

Ken Wilber has espoused an approach to integral practice and development in which we simultaneously include a range of different practices in our self-development. As he says in *One Taste* (1999, p77–78):

> [A]nybody can put together their own integral practice. The idea is to simultaneously exercise all the major levels and dimensions of the human bodymind — physical, emotional, mental, social, cultural, spiritual.... Pick a basic practice from each category, or from as many categories as pragmatically possible, and practice them concurrently – all-level, all-quadrant... In short, exercise body, mind, soul, and spirit in self, culture, and nature.

Working on our personal development can also be part of our everyday lives and work without engaging in any special activity, to the extent we might bring awareness and self-reflection to what we are doing, experiencing and learning. Clearly this is more likely to be true for some professions and types of work than others. Coaching is obviously a profession that is suited to people who are interested in their own personal development and the central theme of this chapter is that developing as a psychosynthesis coach and engaging in your own personal development are mutually supportive and interdependent. One of the amazing things about the coaching profession is that it provides continuing opportunities for the coach to further their own personal development – we need never stop learning from coaching our clients. However, we still need to give time and space to the self-reflective process in which we make meaning for ourselves, which is why supervision is so important for the coach and can be as much about your personal development as your professional practice. For myself, in this phase of my life, the most fruitful form of personal development seems to be working to support the personal and professional development of others, as a teacher, facilitator, coach and supervisor. And yet I notice the need to be in individual and group supervision relationships in which the roles are reversed.

Finding your edges to work on – this tricky part of personal development

In my experience one of the hardest parts of personal development is identifying and focusing on the psychological issues and personality edges that I need to work on. This is because the nature of the issues means they can be elusive and slippery, with our minds unwilling to acknowledge or remember them because they are part of our ingrained and unconscious survival strategies. This work links with the theme of transforming mindsets, which I have written about elsewhere and which is developed in more detail in Chapter 15. This is different to creating a broad vision for one's personal development and setting high-level developmental objectives (which is important but relatively easy) although these two levels of focusing can and should inform each other.

A few approaches come immediately to mind. The first, and probably easiest, is journaling, writing down your thoughts either in the moment as they come or as a regular discipline, for example daily or weekly. The second, rather obviously, is to use coaching to talk through the edges and issues you want to work on with someone else. Sometimes we expect people to come to coaching with their goals or the issues they want to work on fully formed – whereas surfacing these can be the first, and often most important, part of coaching. As a coach I have often worked with leaders to simply reflect upon, unpack and make sense of the most troubling or problematic situations and relationships they have experienced since the previous coaching session and, in most organisations, these are usually plentiful. The key here is the depth of self-reflection and the willingness of the coachee to focus on the part they have played in the problems they experience. A third approach is to use some form of formal or informal feedback exercise alongside personality or leadership profiling.

Assessing your personal development

How might we assess our personal development? Self-reflection, drawing on our own subjective experience, is the cornerstone for any self-assessment. This is best supported by keeping a learning journal and through periodic discussion with a coach. On our courses we ask students to keep a journal and at the end of three months to write a paper reflecting upon their personal and professional development during the course. Any self-assessment is enhanced by setting well-formed, developmental objectives and reviewing progress periodically against these, again ideally with the help of a coach. This can be supported by the use of 360 feedback and personality profiling exercises and this is an approach I use with many of the leaders I coach.

How about assessing the personal development of others – the people we are coaching, for example? In Chapter 11, on leadership development, we make the distinction between horizontal, vertical and inner development, and each of these perspectives lends itself to a different assessment approach. **Horizontal development** mostly concerns abilities, competencies and skills, and there are well-established approaches to assessing these within the organisational human resources world. Increasingly, personal development is playing a more prominent role in leadership development: competency frameworks, emotional intelligence (EQ) and now social intelligence (see Daniel Goleman's work for some useful assessment tools). **Vertical development** is less straightforward, in that a 'paper' self-assessment of vertical development isn't always reliable and 360 feedback is problematic if assessors are less vertically developed than the person being assessed. Harthill's Leadership Development Framework (Rooke and Torbert, 2005), which involves sentence completion analysis by experts, is the most widely accepted approach to this and it provides a helpful starting point. Leadership coaches need to develop their own capacity to assess and evaluate the vertical development of their coachees and there is work to be done to support this. **Inner development,** which is the core development of self and will, building our awareness and capacity to act expressed both in terms of horizontal and vertical development, is even harder to assess, and I would suggest is best grounded in the coach's subjective awareness and observation.

Let me elaborate on what I mean by this. Something I notice when I start coaching a new leader is my automatic and unconscious tendency to formulate a view of their level of self-awareness and ability to self-reflect as being the most significant indicator of their inner development. For example I assess how easy it is to start to create an aware relational space with them. I then start looking for signs of how aware they are of others and the differences in people, as well as recognition of how they impact others. I am wary of coachees telling stories about problems they have with others in their lives that do not include some awareness of their part in it. I might also start to assess how aware they are of the bigger picture they are part of and the systems forces that are impacting them. Can they see and respond systemically to what is going on or are they the unwitting victim? Alongside the leader's levels of awareness (of self, others and the wider system), I am also looking for indications of their capacity to act in the world and the availability of free will in their lives. This tends to take longer to assess and comes partly from seeing evidence of acting upon the realisations, choices and decisions that take place in the coaching space. Finally, I am interested in their attitude and openness to learning (as described in the first point in this piece) and their willingness to ask for help where appropriate. Can they invite and be open to feedback? Can they show any vulnerability or are they too well-defended? The more senior the leader, the more wary I might be of the egotistic or hubristic leader, who knows it all and can do it all.

I have just described the five dimensions of a developmental model that can be used as a way of gauging inner leadership development. This is Roger Evans' 5DL (Five Dimensions of Leadership) model (2020), which is more fully elaborated in Chapter 11, along with Evans's approach to scoring self and others along these five dimensions. For now, here is a quick summary:

1DL – Ability to self-reflect – self-awareness

2DL – Awareness of one's impact on others, understanding their difference and their group dynamics

3DL – Ability to consistently see the whole picture and the dynamics between the 'part and the whole'. The art of 'thinking systemically' and understanding system forces.

4DL – Free will, individual freedom to make clear decisions and to deliver in the face of resistance – 'to be blown in the wind, to bend but to stand firm'

5DL – Ability to ask for appropriate help and support – internally and externally to the organisation. Humanity, humility and openness to feedback.

Knowing it's always personal

Being a coach is always both personal and professional, especially so for psychosynthesis coaches. It is personal in that we can never leave ourselves out of the picture in our reflective professional practice – our subjective experience is the ever-present filter through which we engage in the professional relationship, so paradoxically in order to achieve some degree of objectivity in our perspective, we need to be ever attentive, curious and inquiring about who and how we are, about what is going on with us in relationship to the other. Beyond this, as coaches, we are also always learning about how to use the self as an instrument of change – and there is more scope to be actively and personally engaged in the coaching relationship than in therapy (see Millichamp, 2018), at the same time as always maintaining the context of the professional helping relationship.

Chapter 8

The full model of psychosynthesis coaching

What is our full model of psychosynthesis coaching? What is the context and method of psychosynthesis coaching? What are the key models, tools and skills?

Introduction

Coaching as a professional activity involves holding a **context**, following a **method** or **process**, working with client **agendas**, making **interventions** and drawing upon **skills**. These are the essential, irreducible elements of professional coaching. A full and comprehensive model of coaching should address all these aspects; otherwise I have found that the inexperienced coach will tend to fill in the blanks, either drawing from their previous experience or upon unconscious or unexamined assumptions.

Therefore, in addition to the core psychosynthesis model, I will elaborate other key models which are needed by coaches relating to coaching process, coaching agendas, coaching interventions and coaching skills. I will show how these come together into a dynamic whole for the psychosynthesis coach.

Coaching context and method: trifocal vision and the six-session model

The underlying context for all psychosynthesis coaching work that involves others, whether leaders, individuals, groups or the whole system, is trifocal vision, as developed by Roger Evans for the Institute of Psychosynthesis. Trifocal vision is first referred to by Roberto Assagioli in *The Act of Will* (1974, p184):

> it may be said that trifocal vision is required; that is the perception and retention in mind of the distant goal and purpose; the survey of the intermediate stages which extend from the point of departure to the arrival; and the awareness of the next steps to be taken.

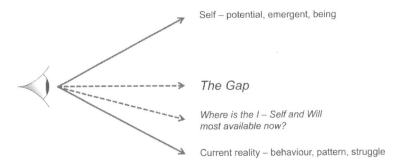

Self – potential, emergent, being

The Gap

Where is the I – Self and Will most available now?

Current reality – behaviour, pattern, struggle

Figure 8.1 Trifocal vision.
Adapted from material by Roger Evans, Institute of Psychosynthesis (2015).

He reminds us that *every phase has its most favourable, even its only possible, moment of execution*. Roger Evans has gradually extended and adapted this concept to the practice of coaching, building upon the concept of bifocal vision which is used in psychosynthesis counselling and therapy.

The following extract, adapted by Paul Elliott for PCL from Institute of Psychosynthesis training material (2015), elaborates our understanding, as illustrated in Figure 8.1:

> What we are saying as we hold and work with Trifocal Vision is that the person is a Self in potential. So there is both this self in potential (that which he/she aspires to be) and there is also his/her personal/work life, as it is today (hence bifocal), mediated through his/her personality (which is the sum total of how this person has learned to function in the world).
>
> This concept of Trifocal Vision enables the coach to hold both the potential of the other person as well as the reality of how they act and behave now. The gap between the reality and the potential is often large and experienced as too hard, too difficult or painful.
>
> How coaches work to manage the process of dealing with (or bridging) this gap is the core substance of psychosynthesis coaching.

More from our PLC material adapted by Paul Elliott on working in the gap:

> Critical to the process of bridging the gap is to help the coachee get some sense of the next realistic and realisable step that will move her/him along the continuum from what is now towards her/his potential. These steps need to be big enough to be challenging and small enough to be achievable. So we see step 1, step 2, step 3 et al. – each step becoming a context for the next level of work.

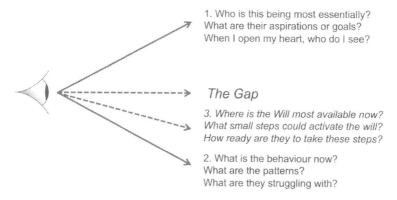

1. Who is this being most essentially?
What are their aspirations or goals?
When I open my heart, who do I see?

The Gap

3. Where is the Will most available now?
What small steps could activate the will?
How ready are they to take these steps?

2. What is the behaviour now?
What are the patterns?
What are they struggling with?

Figure 8.2 Trifocal vision questions.
Adapted from material by Roger Evans, Institute of Psychosynthesis (2015).

The thrust of the work over time is to help the coachee develop his/ her own inner skills of personal mastery and thereby learn to manage the gap. We are seeking to help our clients find where their will is most available and start to make the changes they want to make.

Trifocal context questions (see Figure 8.2) that we might reflect upon include (adapted from material by Roger Evans, Institute of Psychosynthesis, 2015):

Where is the emergent Self? Conscious and unconscious symptoms and signs?

Where is the coachee now? Where is their sense of self and how well formed is their will?

What is the gap and how do we work with it? Where is the will available?

An important difference between this approach and most conventional coaching is the way the coach holds the struggle and the symptoms the coachee is presenting within the context of Self, as summarised by Roger Evans and Paul Elliott in Joan Evans et al. (2013), p201:

The theory and practice of psychosynthesis coaching rests upon the idea that Self is always seeking to express itself; speaking through the client's symptoms – the difficulties and suffering experienced in the personality, which brings them to coaching – is the urge to wholeness, to expression and realisation of Self.

Six-session model

Roger Evans emphasises the importance of combining trifocal vision with a coaching method or process that holds an overall goal for a series of six sessions. His approach breaks this down into individual session goals, which in turn helps focus the coachee on the most appropriate next steps to take towards their goal.

Again, from our (PCL) material adapted by Paul Elliott, from Institute material (2015):

> The gap between where the coaching client is and where they want to be is where we are working. But the gap is usually too wide and it is not possible to get there in one or two sessions. We need to find where their will is most available. So the way of working is to identify the overall goal for a series of 6 one or two-hour sessions. Each session works on a small goal which coach and client agree is important to achieving the overall goal.

We therefore break down larger goals into smaller goals and steps and also recommend that these sessions take place at two-weekly intervals, although some organisations prefer to work on a monthly cycle. Weekly sessions can also be appropriate for dealing with crises, but at other times will be too intense, without enough time between sessions for the client to act in the world. You also might initially contract for a longer period than three months and then continue working with a client through a number of six-session cycles according to their needs. Although the way that sessions are packaged within a contract can obviously vary according to many situational factors, the six-session model is our recommended starting point.

Right relations model

The right relations model, as developed for the Institute of Psychosynthesis by Danielle Roux (see Figure 8.3), helps orientate the coach towards the creation of a being space with their coaching client and guides them in holding the being of the other in a qualitatively different way to how we engage in most of our day-to-day relationships. We introduce the model on the first weekend of our PGCPLC course, using an exercise to develop skills of deeper listening (with the whole being in the here and now), and we invariably observe a shift taking place for the practising coaches in their awareness and contact with the other in the exercise. We have found this to be a key step in helping the student coach to internalise and start to practise trifocal vision in their coaching.

In my experience, holding trifocal vision and seeing the being of the other takes much practice as a coach, as we drift in and out of holding it, forget entirely about it as we are caught in the flow and draw upon it reflectively outside of the coaching session. This is where coaching supervision plays a

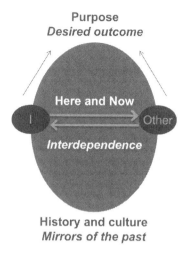

Purpose
Desired outcome

Here and Now

I ⟷ Other

Interdependence

History and culture
Mirrors of the past

Figure 8.3 The right relations model.

very important role. The capacity to hold trifocal vision grows over time and gradually becomes more automatic.

Trifocal vision is what essentially distinguishes and elevates this from other approaches. Combined in practice with the six-session model and supported by right relations skills, it comprises the core of the model of psychosynthesis coaching.

Coaching process model

For the psychosynthesis-trained practitioner (that is, someone who has studied psychosynthesis for two years or more with the Institute or another school) who is approaching coaching for the first time, trifocal vision with the six-session model may provide sufficient method for them to follow in their coaching practice. So far we have focused on how trifocal vision provides a context for holding the client. In a practical method or process, the coach shifts attention between herself and her client, asking the client questions about the three parts in focus, about the emergent Self as expressed in a goal or purpose, about the current reality and where they are now and about the gap and where the will is most available. The coach works with the client to identify and commit to small steps they can take towards their goal. There are many subtleties and nuances to be negotiated as the coach shifts their attention between inner awareness or reflection and outer exploration with the client, through asking questions and listening.

However, I have found that some new coaches need a more explicit process model to work with in coaching, something that provides a simple handrail that they can follow or fall back on in the coaching session. Experienced coaches may already be using such a coaching process. I have therefore found it useful to look at how Trifocal vision can be used in conjunction with a more explicit process model. The most commonly used coaching process in both life and leadership coaching today is Sir John Whitmore and Graham Alexander's GROW (Goal, Reality, Options, Will) model. There are others, such as Peter Hawkins' CLEAR model, which corresponds fairly closely to GROW, and Solutions Focus, but I will leave these aside here. I have found GROW can be used as an outer-focused process for asking questions of the client, alongside the self-reflective inner context-holding of Trifocal vision by the coach. In this combination, the elements of GROW are subservient to and follow the elements of Trifocal vision: we hold the Self or being of the other as we ask questions about their goal; we become curious about where they are now as we ask questions about the current reality; we hold a sense of the gap as we ask questions about their options; we look for where the will is available as we ask questions about their will.

The principles of the GROW model, from *Coaching for Performance* (2017), as summarised by Paul Elliott for PCL workshops, are as follows:

- *Establish rapport with client/coachee, active listening and mirroring*
- *Explore with client building awareness and responsibility*
- *Use open questions to build awareness*
- *Create a dynamic model rather than a linear one*
- *Focus after exploration on what next? What will you do? – taking responsibility to make change*
- *Check out readiness for responsibility using scaling*
- *Explore success/failure in subsequent sessions, building awareness and taking responsibility for next steps*

These are all consistent with the model of Trifocal vision. What I find most useful from GROW, however, is the simple focus on asking questions. I offer as illustration the following GROW questions that I have captured from my own practice, which other coaches may find help them formulate their own questions:

Goal + Purpose

- *What do you want from coaching? Why do you want coaching? What do you want from me as a coach?*
- *What do you want from this session? How do you want me to be with you? What would you like to achieve from today?*
- *What overall goal do you have or outcome do you want from our (six) sessions?*
- *How do you want to use this session? Where do you want to start?*
- *Can you rephrase that as a goal or objective?*

Reality + Unpacking

- *What's happened since we last met?*
- *Tell me the story. Tell me more (about that).*
- *What are your reflections on what happened?*
- *What else is going on? What's your part in that?*
- *Is there a pattern here?*

Options + Exploring

- *What are your possible ways forward?*
- *What are some of the options open to you?*
- *What are your opportunities here?*
- *What resources are available to you? Your own? Your relationships? Inside and outside your organisation?*
- *How feasible are these options? How will you assess them? How will you choose one?*

Will + Action

- *How can you move this forward?*
- *What could be your first step?*
- *How ready are you?*
- *What could get in the way?*
- *What will you do? Will you commit to that?*

Coaching agendas model

We are using the term *agenda* synonymously with *issue*, *topic* or *area* to work on. We use agenda because it seems to be the most widely used such term in the field of executive coaching.

One might hold the view that coaching is neutral as to which agendas the client brings – they can bring any issues, needs, purposes, goals or outcomes they want to work on. So why would a coach need a model of agendas?

First of all, I have come across coaches who have quite fixed ideas about what agendas might be valid for coaching – for example that coaching needs to be performance-oriented and directed towards measurable external goals. In this context, an agendas model can be liberating for the coach.

Second, it may be interesting for the coach to reflect upon the nature of the agendas their client brings and how this informs them about their client. For example some clients may focus exclusively on practical outer agendas and others on very personal inner agendas. A key step in developing the client's capacity to self-reflect is to help them move between inner and outer worlds and to see the connections: for example to see the part played by their personality in creating significant outcomes in their life. The coach can also periodically review the journey they have travelled with their client and be curious about what this is telling them. A model of agendas provides the coach with a map of the full territory that they might encounter – and as a psychosynthesis coach this can be very extensive. This can be useful for the coach's long-term development as they learn to become more comfortable and competent with different types of agenda.

Thirdly, a model of agendas helps the coach to broaden their awareness before working to focus on and agree coaching goals with the client (e.g. an overall goal for a series of six sessions and individual goals or desired outcomes for each session). Holding a map of the client's agendas (whether explicit or implicit) also helps to create a context for the goals that a client wants to work on and might be referred back to periodically as part of reviewing or refining coaching goals.

Figure 8.4 presents our PCL model of coaching agendas:

The **agendas** and issues that leaders bring to coaching have both an outer and an inner dimension.

So, how do we describe the *nature and the scope* of the work that takes place with a coach in an inclusive and expansive way, that then allows for specific emphasis to be made by different approaches to coaching (as well as differing between coaching and counselling or therapy)?

In psychosynthesis coaching, we make the distinction between the client's inner and outer worlds and agendas that they might bring to coaching. Alongside this, we can map the different temporal domains of past, present and future, with a further distinction between near and far future.

Below we map out the territory more explicitly using these distinctions:

In simple terms, we might expect conventional behavioural coaching to lean to the right-hand side/outer world and counselling/therapy to the left-hand side/inner world and to focus more on the past than the future. As psychosynthesis coaches, we seek to hold awareness of all these domains. We are open and free to work across them as needed as we follow the coaching

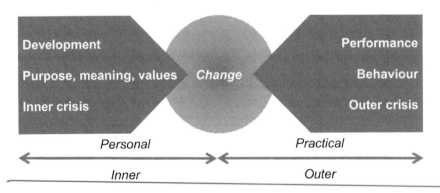

Figure 8.4 The PCL model of coaching agendas.

Table 8.1 The territory of coaching

Orientation and domain	Inner world and agendas/ Being	Outer world and agendas/ Doing
Past	Healing Trauma, reflection, understanding (pre-personal)	Resolution Sense making, acceptance, completion
Present	Inner crisis and change Self, personality, awareness (personal)	Outer crisis and change Systems, relationships, solutions
Near future	Personal development Will, capacity, growth	Performance development Behaviours, skills, actions
Far future	Self-realisation Purpose, meaning, values (transpersonal)	Self-actualisation Potential, career, leadership

process, guided by the four Cs: the context we hold, the contract we establish, the client's needs and issues and our capability and skills.

However, it is extremely important to add that our capability and effectiveness to work across these domains is predicated on drawing upon a core coaching psychology (or combination of psychologies) that is holistic – one that enables practitioners to work with both the inner and outer lives of their clients, navigating the past, present and future. This translates into pre-personal, personal and transpersonal levels, which are embraced within psychosynthesis psychology.

Coaching interventions model

One way of viewing what we do in coaching is as a series of interventions (see Figure 8.5). By intervention, we mean *'an identifiable piece of verbal and/or non-verbal behaviour that is part of the practitioner's service to the client'* (Heron, 1992).

I was first introduced to John Heron's Six Category Intervention Analysis model as part of my first coach training on the MSc Change Agent Skills and Strategies in 1995, and I continue to find this model valuable in the training and development of coaches – to increase awareness of intervention style, develop intervention skills and increase capacity for making different kinds of intervention. Most importantly, the model is useful in challenging a commonly held assumption amongst coaches that all interventions we make should be facilitative. The model shows that there are a range of both authoritative (prescriptive, informative, challenging) and facilitative (cathartic, catalytic, supportive) interventions, which can all be drawn upon according to the needs of the situation. Heron explains that skilful intervention occurs when the intention of the practitioner is congruent with the impact on the client,

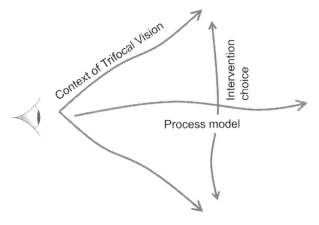

Figure 8.5 The full psychosynthesis coaching model – context, process and intervention.

which involves the choice of intervention type and skill in delivery. However, this is a generic model and is not specific to psychosynthesis coaching, so I will not unpack it in any more detail within this chapter.

Interventions can be viewed at both (i) the micro or granular level (as in Heron's model), which helps us with awareness and skills relating to all our coaching conversations, and (ii) a more macro level, as we consider the options available to us from a more strategic perspective. In my experience, this mostly concerns looking for ways to help the client open up and explore their issues at greater depth – to support awareness and choice in relation to their patterns of behaviour and ability to bring about change in their lives. Within psychosynthesis coaching, I want to highlight three types of intervention we can make to create greater insight for supporting developmental challenges and behavioural change (see Figure 8.6). These are (i) facilitating **mindset** change, (ii) identifying and unpacking **subpersonalities**, and (iii) assessing **leadership styles** and developmental challenges.

These can all be viewed as *different ways in* to working at greater depth and they can be seen as alternative perspectives on the same set of personality and behavioural issues. A mindset (or collection of mindsets) can correspond to a subpersonality, and constellations of mindsets and subpersonalities can be looked at as ways in which archetypal leadership styles are expressed. Thus, the coach can move between working with mindsets, subpersonalities and leadership dimensions depending upon what works best with the individual client. I find that I choose one of these three intervention approaches depending upon cues provided by the client. If the client speaks about their different parts (e.g. 'one part of me thinks this, another part of me thinks that...') this suggests a subpersonalities approach might resonate. If they are prone to unconsciously express strongly held mindsets in relation to

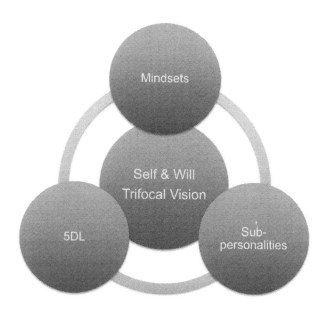

Figure 8.6 Three interventions within the context of trifocal vision.

the issues they are exploring (e.g. 'I can't trust anyone here to get the job done') I might suggest working with a mindset change approach. If they are expressing the issue in the language of leadership behaviours and styles (e.g. 'I want to be more collaborative, but I find it difficult to let go of control...') then I might suggest a leadership styles profiling or 360 feedback exercise as a way of increasing their awareness. The important thing when working with any of these interventions is to remember that they are not an end in themselves – they are subservient to working with the Self and Will of the client and, as such, we are always holding trifocal vision as the context for any of these interventions. Some coaches, and indeed clients, can get carried away with subpersonality work as a way of recognising, organising and directing one's inner resources. However, what we are ultimately seeking to do is help develop the client's sense of self and I–Self connection, alongside a capacity for free will.

Our approach to leadership styles is fully explained in Chapter 13. In Chapter 15, on working with change, I will provide some explanation of the way we work with mindsets and subpersonalities.

Coaching skills model

For purposes of coach development, psychosynthesis coaching also needs an explicit model of coaching skills or competencies. In 2014 I reviewed the ICF competencies model (see Chapter 1), which is the most commonly referred to in the coaching world, and concluded it lacked coherence and consistency; it seems an ad-hoc mix of generic human and communication skills, along with practical or process-related coaching skills, without any guiding logic. I therefore developed our own coaching competencies model for PCL, which acts as a reference for the programme and for participants' continuing personal and professional development as coaches. This makes key distinctions between core *human* skills (which are transferable from a wide range of development contexts including leadership development), core *process* skills (which are transferable from other organisational practitioner and helping professions) and *meta* skills (which are largely transferable from psycho-spiritual practitioner development). This is expanded below:

Human skills

1   Listening with the being
2   Powerful questioning
3   Dynamic communication
4   Building trust in the coaching alliance
5   Impact and influence
6   Right relationships

Process skills

1   Engagement and contracting
2   Creating awareness
3   Agenda forming and goal setting
4   Planning interventions
5   Managing the coaching process
6   Reviewing progress

Meta skills

1   Self-reflection, as the foundation for reflective practice
2   Presence and being authentic
3   Psycho-spiritual mindedness
4   Mastery of the psychological functions, including imagination and intuition
5   Using Self/self as an instrument of change
6   Systemic thinking, holding multiple perspectives, working at different levels

This framework more than adequately covers the coaching competencies identified by the International Coaching Federation. Where possible,

I have used the same language as in the ICF framework, to help show correspondence.

The only meta-skill that is included in the ICF framework is *Presence*. We would expect the human skills and the process skills to be fairly consistent across different approaches to coaching. Meta skills are where the psychosynthesis coach becomes gradually more differentiated, both from more behaviourally oriented approaches and from other coaching psychologies. The cornerstone to meta-skills is the capacity for *Self-reflection* (see DL1 in Evans' *Five Dimensions of Leadership*). *Presence and being authentic* and *Using self as an instrument of change* are meta-skills which might be found in common with other psychological approaches such as Gestalt. *Psychospiritual mindedness* and *Mastery of the psychological functions* are where the psychosynthesis coach becomes most differentiated, developing the capacity to think psycho-spiritually and to exercise the will in relationship with psychological functions such as thinking and feeling, as well as imagination and intuition. Finally, *Systemic thinking* (see DL3 in Evans' *Five Dimensions of Leadership*) is an important differentiator in leadership coaching, both to deal with the complexities of organisational life and to navigate between different levels of working in leadership coaching. Incidentally, DL2 is addressed within the scope of the human skills, particularly *Impact and influence* and *Right relations*. We will unpack Evans' *Five Dimensions of Leadership* more fully in Chapter 8 as our key model of leadership development, but first we will address some important boundary issues and distinctions concerning coaching in general and psychosynthesis coaching in particular.

A coaching story: *Becoming more strategic*

Tony's leadership 360 review had given him some uneven feedback. He was highly rated by his own team and much appreciated by his colleagues for the energy, qualities and skills he brought to the leadership team (which matched with his own self-evaluation), but consistently scored lower in all categories by his manager. After the feedback session with the coach, Tony had spent some serious time reflecting on all the feedback and the changes he wanted to bring about for himself. He knew he needed to become less focused on day-to-day operational priorities and more strategic in his role as marketing director, and this meant some major changes to the way he worked.

At the next session, Tony unpacked the key changes he had decided to make, including learning to delegate better, improving his own communication (especially upline), creating more space for strategic work and checking out his intuitions with others. He and the coach worked together on what each of these meant and what steps Tony could take towards them. The coach then guided Tony to think about the under-lying psychological patterns and personality edges that held the old behaviours in place. At the end, Tony reflected: 'I'm very disciplined but can also be too hard on myself. Perhaps I need to lighten up and free-wheel a bit. I could trust the process more and be less task led'.

At the next session Tony revealed the breakthrough started by the previous session and the brainstorm that had followed. By increasing his awareness of his personal psychology (or how he got caught by his edges, as the coach described it), he was able to depersonalise (or disidentify and witness, as the coach described it) from the systemic issues and forces within the organisation, which allowed him to more freely establish and follow his own personal strategies and disciplines (or activate his free will, as the coach described it), which include man-aging his own energy and space (and to build his sense of self and resili-ence, as the coach described it).

There was still the big disparity in his manager's feedback to deal with. At the next session, the coach encouraged Tony to set up a one-to-one to with his boss, to find out more of his thinking behind the feedback. This took place and the conversation brought clarity, understanding and a closer working relationship. The organisation was going through some big changes following a takeover, so it was also important that Tony and his boss could speak freely about the opportunities and the best role for Tony in the new set up. In the following session, the coach and Tony explored some of the possible avenues he might follow and how to take the initiative towards his preferred option. The coach helped Tony visualise what this might look like a year from now.

The final sixth session was taken up planning the contribution Tony was going to make at the upcoming leadership team off-site meeting. Tony had taken the initiative to develop a strategic framework to guide the team through the organisational and human change that was needed. The team event was a great success and by the end of the work-shop his manager and colleagues had started to see Tony in a new light. His primary goal of becoming more strategic within his role had been achieved.

Chapter 9

Boundaries, ambiguities and contexts

What distinguishes psychosynthesis leadership coaching from life coaching?

What distinguishes psychosynthesis coaching from therapy?

How might leaders develop their psychosynthesis coaching skills when coaching their people?

Life coaching versus leadership coaching

Below I have set out some key distinctions between leadership coaching and life coaching.

Leadership coaching...

- focuses on leadership as a calling and orientation rather than as a formal role – we can all be leaders to some extent within our roles in work or life in general
- takes place within an organisational and systemic context involving multiple clients; usually this means a coaching sponsor as well as individual coaching clients
- can involve working with individuals and teams as part of an organisational system
- can encompass multiple agendas, issues and goals, including those of performance, behaviour and change, as well as personal development, purpose, meaning and values.

Life coaching...

- takes place within the context of the client's whole life rather than their work or role
- has a sole client, the person who is being coached
- can also encompass many agendas, issues and goals such as work and career, relationships and family, health and finance, change and crisis, personal development, purpose, meaning and values.

As I said in the introduction, in this book I have chosen to focus on leadership coaching. This is partly because that is where my interest, experience and expertise lie, but also because there are tricky issues concerned with life coaching which I would prefer not to enter into here, for example the shifting boundaries with counselling and a lack of clear professional standards required to support the present explosion of people calling themselves life coaches. However, I do want to tackle the more generic issue concerning the relationship between therapy or counselling and any form of coaching, which I do below.

Therapy versus coaching

When running courses on coaching we are frequently asked questions about the relationship, boundaries and differences between therapy, counselling and coaching. This topic is fraught with difficulty and complexity and is prone to trite or superficial treatment, so this section (developed from an article posted on LinkedIn) is intended to shed some light on it.

If you Google 'What is the difference between therapy, counselling and coaching?' or something similar you will find plenty of generally superficial answers seeking to delineate territory that limits the scope of both counselling and coaching to fit the author's agenda (an acknowledgement – I too have an agenda!).

Michael Bader in his article in *Psychology Today,* 'The Difference Between Coaching and Therapy is Greatly Overstated' *(*2009), clearly identifies the problem from stories he often hears from coaches, who say that they work with the future and therapists with the past; that coaches work to make healthy clients better, while therapists work with pathology and problems. He suggests:

> that this is a mythic narrative that aims to insulate coaching – a profession in its infancy – from claims that it's therapy without a license. It seeks to protect the egos and wallets of coaches while appeasing therapists on the same grounds.

He goes on to lay some of the blame for this at the door of the therapy profession for practising 'a model of psychotherapy that is so ridiculously narrow and theory-driven' (ibid.).

A good example of this dodgy narrative can be found on Tony Robbins' website (www.tonyrobbins.com/coaching/) – *life coach vs therapist, learn the difference,* which – although acknowledging overlaps – proceeds to define coaching in very narrow terms of client agendas (e.g. working to improve communication skills or work–life balance) that fit his target market of ambitious achievers (e.g. Laloux's Achievement paradigm).

Even worse offenders (whom I will not name) in perpetuating this dodgy narrative make sweeping distinctions (in addition to the common *future* and *past* delineation), along the lines that coaching deals with the conscious mind, rational behaviours and measurable goals, involves positive thinking and focuses on solutions (i.e. all the good stuff), whereas therapy or counselling works with the unconscious mind, with emotions, subjective goals, pathologies and problems (i.e. all the murky stuff). This narrative is usually espoused by coaching schools that offer a very prescriptive method for young or inexperienced coaches on the basis that if they follow the method this will keep them (and their client) safe from straying off the path or into deep waters. The problem with this very delineated approach (*this* belongs to coaching, *that* belongs to counselling) is that people (i.e. all clients) are whole human beings who bring the good stuff as well as the murky stuff with them, their light and their dark mirrors, their conscious goals and their unconscious drives, whether to coaching or counselling. There is another fundamental problem with any attempt to separate rational and emotional domains – all the recent neuro-psychological research (e.g. Daniel Kahneman's *Thinking Fast and Thinking Slow* (2012)) points towards a much greater role for the unconscious and our emotions in all our behaviour and decision-making than has been previously acknowledged by the modern western worldview. This is particularly clear in business and organisational life where, despite a new awareness slowly emerging, rational and individual agency has been elevated at the expense of the emotional and human system.

Some better approaches (from my Google search) tackle the distinction by working through themes such as the objectives, agendas or focus (of the activity); education, training and qualification (required of practitioners); ethics and governance (of the profession); or approaches and methods (e.g. psychologies) used. The most useful commentary along these lines is one I found on a post by the South African College of Applied Psychology (2014), which describes the relationship between professional counsellors and coaches as comparable to that of step-siblings. The author goes on,

> The emphasis in a coaching relationship is on goals, action and accountability, although an experienced coach will know when to look at the past should it inform the present and help pinpoint limiting belief systems. So while counselling is geared towards understanding and resolving the past so as to promote healing, coaching works with functional people and uses the past only insofar as it provides a context in which future goals can be set.

This goes some way to teasing out the subtleties needed but is still part of a static approach and, as such, has limitations.

In response to this need to differentiate counselling and coaching, I developed the dynamic framework called the Four Cs (Context, Contract, Client and Coach) that I presented in Chapter 1, which can (i) help us understand differences *within* coaching and counselling practice as well as *between* coaching and counselling and (ii) also help coaches and counsellors alike think critically about how they frame and identify boundaries around the work they do.

Coaching supervision

It seems a good place here to lightly touch upon the topic of supervision. Coaching supervision is becoming an established role and field of development in its own right and, with Roger Evans' recently established PGC in psychosynthesis coaching supervision, we now have a recognised path for psychosynthesis coaches and coaching supervisors to follow. The importance for all coaches to have some form of supervision for their practice is becoming widely accepted, although in practise not all coaches do. The principle of mirrored support systems in which each practitioner has a space where they can be held in relationship to and by another, where they can reflect upon and unpack the work they are doing, is also becoming increasingly recognised. It is also seen as providing an important ethical foundation to our professional practice.

Supervision has several possible functions and uses, the emphasis on which may vary according to the needs and level of experience of the coach and the work they are doing with leaders. Psychosynthesis coaching supervision can be used to support coaches to reflect upon their practice and application of trifocal vision in particular. Supervision is also a space to which the coach can take any moral or ethical dilemmas and issues of personal and professional boundaries and, where appropriate, to seek advice or guidance from the supervisor. Thus the coach is always held in a safe professional context that helps establish and maintain the integrity of the coaching in alignment with any code of practice that the coach has made a commitment to. Supervision can also be used to support the coach more broadly in their personal and professional development over time.

Within psychosynthesis coaching supervision, the most important emphasis is to develop the capacity of the coach to self-reflect through guiding and supporting their own self-supervision. As the starting point for this, we use a supervision template, which the coach completes in preparation for a session in relationship to a particular client. The template challenges the coach to reflect using trifocal vision by asking a series of questions, including: *Who do you see when you open your heart to this person? What are they struggling with, or where are they caught? What is the big gap (between the emergent Self and the current reality) that you are working in? Where is the will most available and how might this be activated by taking a small step towards the goal?* Further questions help the coach to describe the coachee's goal (or goals), the next small step towards this and the readiness of the coachee to activate their will. A further section supports the coach's deeper reflections from each session and looks at the series of coaching sessions as a whole. Where appropriate, we add a further section for the coach to assess the coachee according to the 5DL model we introduce in the next chapter. We introduce this supervision template more fully and in its entirety on our leadership coaching courses and with any coaches we are supervising.

A supervisor may shift between modalities within a supervision session – for example between *super-vision, super-coaching, coaching* and *mentoring*. The important thing here, from the perspective of the supervisor, is that they are doing this intentionally, or at least that they are aware of making these shifts and have choice in relation to them. It is also important from the coach's perspective that they are aware of what they need and want from the supervisor and that the way they are working together is congruent with their implicit or explicit contract. *Super-coaching* is when the supervisor steps into the coach's shoes and suggests what to look for or how they might approach the coachee, or gives examples of the questions they might ask. *Coaching* might take place when the coach needs to explore or reflect upon their personal development or psychological edges. *Mentoring* can be appropriate when the supervisor has valuable information or experience to draw from in relation to the situation or circumstances the coach finds themselves in, for example about how a particular sector or organisation works. Mostly though, psychosynthesis *super-vision* should be about supporting the coach's ability to reflect on their coaching and that of their coachees.

For those wishing to explore the role of supervision more fully for themselves, I would highlight Peter Hawkins and Robin Shohet's *Supervision in the Helping Professions* (2012), where they unpack their Seven Eyed Model, as a good starting point. I would also recommend Alison Hodges' paper for APECS, 'How supervision can make a difference' (2015). My own supervisor, Fiona Adamson, is co-authoring a book on supervision drawing upon a transpersonal perspective, which I am greatly looking forward to reading.

Leaders as coaches

This book is primarily addressed to the specialist leadership coach, whether internal or external to an organisation, and towards explicit coaching activity, whether this is a primary or part-time professional activity for the coach. We occasionally make reference to leaders as coaches and I hope that much of this book will be relevant to leaders who want to develop a coaching style of leadership. However, there are many issues and challenges that leaders face when developing a coaching style as part of the way they work that are not touched upon in this book. This is the reverse of the way John Whitmore wrote and positioned *Coaching for Performance* (2017). He is primarily speaking to leaders and managers and secondarily the specialist coach, which helps explain the success of the book, with more than one million copies sold. Whitmore explores some of the issues of the leader as coach in Chapter 4 of his book.

Of course I want to encourage leaders to adopt more of an empowering, facilitative coaching style in the way they lead and manage, rather than an authoritative and directive or micro-management style, because this is likely to lead to empowered people and better results. There are many skills, models and approaches within this book that will support the leader in doing that. Some leaders may also be able to engage with the deeper psychological reflection demanded of the psychosynthesis coach and commit to the personal development journey that this path entails, and this may help them become truly exceptional leaders – but that is the point: they are likely to be the exception. We continue to have small numbers of leaders attending our PGCPLC coaching programmes with the intention purely that they become better leaders in their organisations; in the future, we may develop a version of our programme more specifically designed for leaders as coaches, most likely tailored to different sectors or for a specific organisation.

Using our 4Cs framework, the *context* is entirely different for the leader as coach – they are coaching people who may report to them or over whom they may have some authority, so the realisation of a confidential and safe space for the coaching is very difficult to achieve. There may or may not be a coaching *contract* of some kind, either explicit or implicit, depending upon whether the leader has set a context for the way they are working with the *coachee*. The important thing here is that the leader is aware of the power imbalance in the relationship and that they take this into account when they coach. One quality most people appreciate in a leader is consistency, and it is important that leaders realise this when seeking to shift their management style. The leader who swings between micro-management and coaching may create more confusion than empowerment.

Finally, I would encourage any leaders seeking to develop a coaching style to make sure that they are receiving coaching themselves, ideally with an external specialist coach, but at least with an internal coach with whom they can establish a confidential relationship. This is an essential support to their progress as a leader coach through self-reflective practice and professional development.

Internal coaching

Internal coaching is growing significantly within organisations and in many ways it may be where the future of coaching lies. There are at least two types of internal coach: (i) the specialist professional coach for whom coaching is the primary activity (or maybe part of a portfolio within an organisational development role) and (ii) the part-time or job-plus coach who has a different primary role in the organisation but allocates an agreed part of their time (e.g. one day a month or one day a week) to coaching colleagues with whom they have no direct day-to-day relationship.

Again, it is helpful to use the 4Cs framework to reflect upon some of the boundary and ethical issues of internal coaching vis-à-vis external coaching. The *context* of internal coaching makes it important that coaches and coachees are matched together well (usually by someone in an HR or other central role) so that the coachee can feel safe in the relationship. Additionally, good *contracting* is needed to ensure the coaching continues and is protected from a variety of distractions that may affect both parties. Enlightened organisations will require minimal or no reporting back from the coach to the line manager of the coach, to protect the confidentiality of the coaching sessions.

There are considerable benefits to an organisation for developing a cadre of internal job-plus coaches. These include (i) the direct impact of many more leaders being coached than would otherwise be possible; (ii) the improvement in leadership learning and skills development for the job-plus coaches; (iii) the likely increase in job satisfaction for the job-plus coaches; and (iv) the long term impact of creating a coaching culture as a major organisational development intervention.

My mentor, friend and colleague Anne Welsh recently completed an involvement that had lasted for many years, to establish and support a coaching culture with GlaxoSmithKline (GSK). She led the training and supervision of more than 650 job-plus coaches across the globe, working alongside many other psychosynthesis trained coaches, both those employed by GSK and those working as external executive coaches – including another good friend and colleague, Sue Cruse. The story of coaching in GSK is really for them and others to tell, and I will not attempt to relay it here. Anne ran a session at PCL's recent symposium in February 2020, in which she shared something of both her own story of psychosynthesis and that of coaching at GSK. I hope there will be something we can share more widely coming from this symposium session. I have met many people who have been involved in this endeavour and believe that it provides one of the best examples of the difference that a coaching culture can make within an organisation. Some of the job-plus coaches came to realise that leadership coaching was their calling and made long-term career decisions in this direction, which led them onto our PGCPLC programme. For many others, the experience of being a job-plus coach will have had a lasting beneficial impact upon their capability and success as a leader.

We are already starting to adapt our programmes as in-house coach training for internal and job-plus coaches and my sense is that this will be the largest growth area for coaching over the next ten years or so.

Frederic Laloux, in *Re-inventing Organizations* (2014), tells the story (pages 62–73) of Jos de Block and the organisation called Buurtzorg he created in 2006 for the provision of neighbourhood nursing services in the Netherlands. It was founded on the principle of self-organising teams of ten to twelve nurses with no manager and no team leader: this model worked so well that it quickly grew to provide most of the nursing care services across the country. The central organisation was kept to a minimum, primarily there to share resources, ideas and knowledge between the teams. Of course, problems would sometimes arise in the teams which required outside help and the central organisation set up a team of coaches, each of whom is responsible for supporting a number of neighbourhood teams and who could also provide team facilitation and coaching to help resolve issues and enable creative solutions if required. This is an example of where the role of the internal coach will have almost entirely replaced the role of manager, and I see this as a blueprint for how some organisations might develop in the future.

Chapter 10

Personal and professional
Part 3

> *Everything, every behaviour, is a vibratory pattern or process. Such process emerges, develops and decays, according to a single principle. People have a natural reverence for the principle and they naturally love the vibratory energy which obeys the principle.*
>
> John Heider, *Tao of Leadership* (1985), an adaptation
> of Lao Tzu's *Tao Te Ching*

Part 3: personality and personal development

In Chapter 3 we summarised the primary task of personal development as getting to know and mastering our personality by exploring all levels of our consciousness. This undertaking, both for ourselves and in support of our clients, benefits from having some good maps of the territory. My aim in this chapter is to overview some useful models of personality as well as to contribute something new that might be of value to coaches. At the same time we must remember that any maps are there simply to support the real work of exploration and discovery taking place at the individual level in coaching and other personal development activity. As much as possible I will illustrate how to apply the models using the example of my own personal development journey.

I start with Jung's personality typology and Assagioli's psychological elements, which together provide a fairly comprehensive overview of the territory of the personality. I will then introduce some of the better-known tools for identifying personality issues, before working towards my own model of psychological health that combines (i) individuation – how we are in our relationship with others – with (ii) self-sense – how we are in our relationship with ourselves. It is important to remember that our interest is in exploring the territory of what we call healthy neurosis here rather than pathology, so our perspective is rather different to that of conventional psychology or psychotherapy.

Jung and Assagioli – personality type and psychological functions

The most common approaches to describing or analysing personality are *type* and *trait* theories, of which I will focus on the theory of *psychological types* developed by Carl Jung. Jung's work has been used as the foundation for some of the most commonly used psychometric profiling tools in organisations, including the Myers-Briggs Type Indicator (MBTI), Insights and DISC.

For those of you who are not familiar with the Jungian typology, below is a very basic summary taken from material I was given on my MSc CASS in the 1990s (original source unknown):

The Jungian typology is concerned with individuals' preferences for four cognitive activities and provides a dichotomous scale for each of these activities, as summarised below:

Where you focus your *attention*	–	Extraversion I or Introversion (I)
The way you take in *information*	–	Sensing (S) or Intuition (N)
The way you make *decisions*	–	Thinking (T) or Feeling (F)
How you *deal* with the outer world	–	Judging (J) or Perceiving (P)

People will tend to have a preference towards one or other pole for each of these four scales, which creates 16 different basic combinations or typologies. Each of the 16 types will tend to be associated with different leadership characteristics and styles. If you have completed a Myers-Briggs (or similar) questionnaire and received your profile, you should know what your Jungian typology is (e.g. ESTJ or INFP).

There are many ways and places to find out more about any of the various flavours of the Jungian system and to generate a profile as a way of getting to know yourself better (e.g. by googling MBTI, Insights or DISC etc.). As with most psychometric tools, I find them both frustrating and intriguing in equal measure; frustrating because of the binary way they are presented, often asking you to make choices between seeming opposites, whereas, just as often, I find the answers are 'it depends' or 'neither', as opposed to one or the other. At the same time, there is a value to profiling that comes from the self-recognition and identification with a type or types, which allows you to see yourself more clearly for who you are and how you are, as well as seeing how others who are not your type(s) are different. Although I would not discourage you or your clients from using such tools, rather than getting too hooked on identifying with a type (e.g. I am 7 and 5 on the Enneagram!)

I would encourage you to use them more qualitatively, creatively and flexibly to explore yourself in different ways. For example you could ask yourself *in what ways am I introverted and in what ways am I extroverted? What might it mean to recognise my feeling nature more? In what way might I be suppressing my feelings and limiting my emotional intelligence? What are the implications of my seeming bias towards intuition over sensory information as my source of information about the world?*

Jung's work popularised the trait of extraversion–introversion as a dimension of human personality, although, unfortunately, its use in popular psychology has become distorted into binary types – that is, are you an introvert or an extrovert, do you like to stay in and read a book or go out to socialise? To quote Wikipedia (https://en.wikipedia.org/wiki/Extraversion_and_introversion, accessed 2018):

> Carl Jung and the developers of the Myers–Briggs Type Indicator provide a different perspective and suggest that everyone has both an extraverted side and an introverted side, with one being more dominant than the other. Rather than focusing on interpersonal behaviour, however, Jung defined introversion as an 'attitude-type characterised by orientation in life through subjective psychic contents' (focus on one's inner psychic activity) and extraversion as 'an attitude type characterised by concentration of interest on the external object' (focus on the outside world).

Assagioli also saw introversion and extraversion as useful primary ways of exploring and mapping our personality, for example (Assagioli, 1965, p148):

> As Jung pointed out, an individual may be both introverted and extraverted according to the different psychological functions; for instance, introverted in the feeling function while extraverted in the thinking function.

I find this attitudinal perspective more useful than the now common behavioural focus. As a coach, what do I notice most about the people I am coaching from a psychological or personality perspective? I notice the extent to which they are focused on their inner world and their outer world and whether they are able to include and move between the two. I often encounter clients at both extremes – either where they are so preoccupied with the outer world of doing, with concrete goals and achievement that they find it hard to articulate their inner world – or they are so caught in their inner world that they find it hard to link personal development to observable and measurable achievement and progress in their lives or work. The former situation is more common in leadership coaching with successful leaders who are outer-oriented and reluctant or unable to explore their inner world.

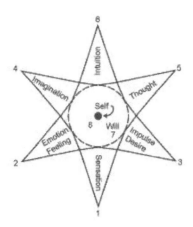

1. Sensation

2. Emotion - Feeling

3. Impulse - Desire

4. Imagination

5. Thought

6. Intuition

7. Will

8. Central point: The I, or personal self

Figure 10.1 Assagioli's star diagram.

Assagioli drew upon Jung's theory of psychological types and added depths and dimensions with his own model of psychological functions. Jung considered there to be four primary psychic functions: sensation, feeling, thought and intuition (250, 1974), to which Assagioli adds **imagination** and **impulse** (or desire). Assagioli importantly places the will and the self at the centre of psychological functioning (see Figure 10.1).

This gives us a map we can work with more dynamically as coaches, with a focus on supporting the healthy engagement and expression of will through mastery of the psychological functions.

Personality issues and edges

FIRO-B is often used to complement Jungian types, with its focus on relational preferences in terms of our needs to express and receive inclusion, control and affection. This can indirectly point towards potential issues to work on, for example where our need to exert structure and control is much greater than our acceptance of structure or control from others (as is the case for myself), but this still needs to be combined with other work such as in coaching in order to personalise the meaning.

I sometimes use the TA Stress Drivers questionnaire as a quick way to help a coachee identify psychological patterns and edges to work on. The five stress drivers are *be perfect; please others; hurry up; try harder;* and *be strong.* The great thing about these is that they are easy to recognise in ourselves, and that everyone will have their own unique stress drivers profile. They also combine well with subpersonalities and mindsets approaches to working with clients. My very strong 'Hurry Up' driver, for example is associated with both

Stage	Neurosis	Remedy
Sensation	*Desensitisation*	Feel
Awareness	*Deflection*	Listen
Energy mobilisation	*Introjection*	Communicate
Action	*Projection*	Own
Contact	*Retroflection*	Engage
Resolution	*Egotism*	Acknowledge
Withdrawal	*Confluence*	Reflect

Figure 10.2 The Gestalt cycle of experience stages with corresponding interruptions and solutions.

my 'rebel' authority-rejecting subpersonality and my mindsets about never having enough time.

Another approach I have drawn upon is the Gestalt cycle of experience (see Figure 10.2), which indicates pathologies that can occur if healthy completion of cycles of experience is interrupted for an individual (also for an organisation). We will tend to form patterns of behaviour in the way that we don't work through complete cycles of experience, and you might recognise points along the cycle below where you get caught and fall into a pattern. For a proper introduction to Gestalt and the cycle of experience within an organisational context I refer you to resources I have made available on our website (www.psychosynthesiscoaching.co.uk/community-resources/).

For example I tend to get caught at the point of *contact* in the cycle of my engagement in the world and instead of ever achieving satisfying *resolutions*, I am onto the next thing that *mobilises my energy*. Recognising this has led me to focus on the need to contain and allow experiences, projects or situations the time and space to come to fruition. I have also increased the attention I give to the start of the cycle – *sensation* and *awareness* – and my ability to respond appropriately to needs arising in my consciousness (whether inner or outer in origin) rather than reacting out of habit or according to outdated patterns.

There are also a number of 'derailer' type approaches (such as Hogan derailers; see: www.hoganassessments.com) which highlight the ways in which leaders trip themselves up through unconscious and unexamined aspects of their personalities (derailers). I have used these on occasion with uneven success – the tools seem too geared towards making the profile analyst or coach seem clever rather than helping the leader or coachee understand themselves better. However, I know many leadership coaches who find these tools a very useful way in to working with the unconscious or shadow side of their clients.

Towards a model of psychological health for coaching

In search of a more accessible map to explain our personality edges or distortions, I turn towards the work of Manfred Kets de Vries (2016) and others who have applied the body of material about attachment theory (following psychoanalyst John Bowlby) to the field of work with organisations and leaders. He suggests that many people, including highly successful leaders and professionals, develop dysfunctional attachment patterns in early life which 'in later life lead to repetitive patterns of unhealthy thoughts and conflictive relationships' (p1). He goes on to describe (ibid.) how:

> More recent works on attachment behaviour propose four attachment styles based upon two dimensions: the **anxiety** dimension – which focuses on the anxiety we may feel about rejection and abandonment – and the **avoidant** dimension – which reflects the discomfort associated with closeness and dependency.

Figure 10.3 below is my attempt to illustrate this, drawing upon Kets de Vries' paper:

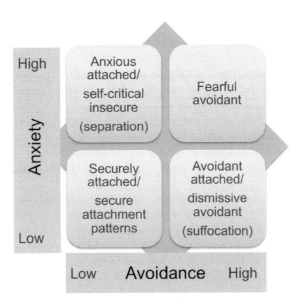

Figure 10.3 Attachment styles, based upon Manfred Kets de Vries (2014).

Gervase Bushe (2010) tackles similar territory by talking in terms of **self-differentiation** patterns, contrasting extremes of fusion and disconnection, which are associated with separation anxiety with suffocation anxiety respectively. The **Fusion** polarity is characterised by too much connection, a lack of boundaries and an over-dependence on what other people think or experience. The **Disconnection** polarity tends towards keeping separate, through maintaining rigid boundaries and not thinking about what others are experiencing (Bushe p80). Bushe goes on to describe the ideal of *self-differentiation*, where we are separate but connected, have choices about boundaries and how we react to others in interactions and want to know what others are experiencing but stay true to our self.

I have added the key terms used by Gervase Bush, *separation* anxiety and *suffocation* anxiety, on the graphic of Kets de Vries' model. On balance, I prefer the language used by Bushe and will adopt his model of **self-differentiation** going forwards as one axis of my overall model of psychological health, i.e. individuation and how we are in relation to others. Bushe's *Clear Leadership* (2010) is the best book I have come across at explaining important psychological ideas in a way that is accessible to the organisational world and I recommend it to leaders, coaches and OD professionals alike.

The psychosynthesis triphasic model of development (developed by Joan Evans and Jarlath Benson; see Simpson and Evans 2014, p21) provides a more detailed and nuanced road map for coaches working to support the differentiation and individuation process. It shows how we are all evolving from *fusion*, to *symbiosis* to *differentiation* at three nested levels – building a strong enough ego, a healthy independent sense of I (as in Bushe's model) and an emergent higher Self. This model is taught on some advanced training programmes in psychosynthesis and we are currently exploring how to apply it more explicitly to coaching.

The second axis of my model of psychological health concerns how we are in our relationship with ourselves – our self-orientation or **self-sense**. One way to think about this dimension is in terms of three separate but inter-related aspects of self-relationship: self-esteem, self-acceptance and self-confidence.

From Wikipedia (article on 'Self-esteem', accessed 2018): **Self-esteem** 'reflects an individual's overall subjective emotional evaluation of his or her own worth... it is the decision made by an individual as an attitude towards the self. Smith et al. (2007, p107) defined it by saying 'The self-concept is what we think about the self; self-esteem, is the positive or negative evaluations of the self, as in how we feel about it'.

Rational Emotive Behavioural Therapy advocates **self- (and other-) acceptance** as a healthier and more useful alternative notion to self-esteem. Self-acceptance is an easier and cleaner attitudinal muscle for the coach to help the coachee focus on than self-esteem, which has the potential to activate unconscious judgements and criticisms, whether about self of others. In this way, practising self-acceptance (and holding compassion for yourself) can be seen as an antidote to low self-esteem.

Self-confidence can be seen as an outcome or consequence of self-esteem and self-acceptance. As coaches, we are more overtly focused on self-confidence in terms of our coachees' willingness and ability to act and take steps towards their goals. Coaching is intimately concerned with building self-confidence for the coachee over time, and the coach is probably holding some awareness of their clients' self-confidence much of the time they are working together.

Low self-esteem is increasingly common in a world in which we are constantly judging or comparing ourselves to others both consciously and unconsciously in different ways. Ego-inflation or excessive self-esteem is less common in the general population but is not unusual in very senior and successful leaders. Most coaches and the people we find ourselves coaching are likely to lean towards the low side of self-esteem or self-confidence. Much of the time in coaching those we call 'healthy neurotics', we are working with a deficiency of self-esteem, self-acceptance or self-confidence, or all three. Sometimes this needs to be worked with directly and explicitly; at other times the experience of exercising and developing the Will and the achievement of stretch goals naturally builds self-confidence.

The ego-inflated leader is less likely to ask for coaching in the first place. The more extreme the case of inflation, the more likely it is to be holding a shadow of insecurity and low self-esteem that often appears on the rebound (what psychoanalysts call negative inflation). The relationship between ego-inflation and narcissism is complex, and although they often come together they can also be found separately. The topic of the narcissistic leader is important if you are working with the most senior leaders and is explored fully by Kets de Vries in his excellent *Leader on the Couch* (2006).

I am not trying to present myself as an expert on these psychological concepts, and there are sources and courses which you can access to build a deeper understanding of them. My purpose here is to provide an overview of the territory and introduce useful concepts for you to work with as a coach in relationship to yourself and the people you are coaching. The point here is to be able to recognise general personality types, leanings and inclinations that help us get to grips with the psychological issues and edges we need to work with in personal development. With this in mind, I will now put the two dimensions together, our relationship to ourselves and our relationship to others, which gives us the **model of psychological health** depicted in Figure 10.4.

The model is dynamic in a number of ways which can't be easily depicted in a two-dimensional graphic.

1   We are interested in a person's *pattern* in relationship to each axis, not just their relative position on a scale. For example we might ask if there is a pattern of movement that swings from one extreme to another, or is there

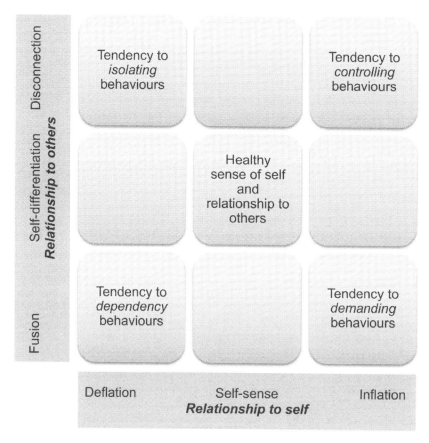

Figure 10.4 Model of psychological health.

relative stability at one place along the axis? Kets de Vries' attachment model shows the possibility of the Fearful–Avoidant pattern, in which an individual is caught in a tension between the polarities of Fusion and Disconnection (e.g. they desperately need people's approval but at the same time feel suffocated by them).

2   In relationship to self the pattern of swinging between deflation and inflation is relatively common and familiar. In extreme cases this might take us into the territory of the bipolar disorder; however, many people experience swing patterns without being bipolar and, frequently, self-esteem can be seen to be contingent on stimulus and events, leading to a 'boom or bust' pattern. We can swing from one polarity to another, for example from feeling energised and purposeful to empty and despondent, but rarely resting in a centred or grounded place between the two. This

can be compounded by the stresses, pressures and anxieties we experience in our lives and work that can make us feel like we are always trying to get somewhere rather than be where we are. This describes a common phenomenon which I will call the 'missing middle' that I recognise both in myself from certain times in my life and in some of my coachees. This state of being calls for work on finding our centre, our ground of being, a place less contingent on the events and outcomes of our daily life. Again we expand on this theme below.

3   The two axes or dimensions are related and interdependent in ways that we won't be able to fully explore here. In other words, the nature of our relationship with others is both informed by and informs the nature of our relationship with ourselves. As a coach, you might intuitively decide which axis needs to be worked on as the priority and then, over time, observe how this work brings about progress on the other axis.

4   In the four corners of the model, I have indicated examples of behavioural tendencies that you might observe in yourself or your coachees. In this way you could use the model to identify in which direction to look for psychological patterns, edges and issues. At the same time, distinguishing three zones on each axis rather than just two polarities gives rise to a healthy central space (healthy self-sense and relationship to others), which we can use as an individualised ideal to work towards and strengthen for ourselves or our coachees.

5   The model doesn't recognise the social, cultural or systemic context within which the individual exists. As already suggested, low self-esteem is becoming a systemic societal issue, particularly amongst young people. The pace and stresses of life are making it increasingly challenging for all of us to stay centred or grounded, which in part has given rise to the current widespread interest in mindfulness practices. This issue could be explored from a social and systemic perspective, but that is beyond my scope here.

6   This is an embryonic model, which needs further development and refinement. I have proposed it because I have not been able to find anything suitable elsewhere in the psychological field. I would welcome an approach from anyone interested in collaborating to validate and develop the model further.

Much of the personal development work in relationship to the theme of self-sense is about building a stronger centre, an experience of groundedness, an ability to be present to ourselves and others, as well as building greater resilience in the face of life's difficult situations, unexpected events and unwelcome influences and the emotions these trigger that take us away from our centre and our ground of being. There are many approaches to this (some of which I named earlier), of which mindfulness and meditation are currently very popular. The causes of our lack of centre or groundedness can be more deep-seated, however, and can usefully be explored within the coaching context. Psychosynthesis offers various approaches to working at different levels of consciousness and development, including the triphasic model referenced earlier.

The practice of **disidentification** is very important in psychosynthesis as a way of building our centre and ground. We can become over-identified with parts of ourselves or the contents of our consciousness and need to work on recognising when this happens and how it affects us and takes us away from our experience of being. Most generally, we can lean towards over-identification with our **body**, our **feelings** or our **mind** (BFM), and then with specific aspects within each of these areas. For example in my long-term personal development I have been working on my primary over-identification with *mind* and my tendency to control my world through thinking. I have experienced myself 'in my head' too much of the time and have found it hard to stay centred and grounded in my being. When I started my psychosynthesis journey, my personal development goal was the resolution of what I experienced as an essential split between my mind and my heart. I will return to continue with this example below.

There is a further dimension to our developing sense of self used within psychosynthesis that is important here. As described in the first chapter of the book, this is our connection with our higher or transpersonal Self, the I-Self connection. It is the territory Assagioli termed *spiritual* or *transpersonal* psychosynthesis and is the second part of our personal development journey.

Trauma and personality splits

The above model is a way of considering our psychological health in terms of our *generalised* relationship with others and with ourselves. It is designed to help the coach recognise the underlying and prevailing personality issues and edges they might be dealing with. We emphasise that our patterns in relationship to the model (swings between polarities, situational variations, etc.) can be many and varied depending upon other psychological and personality factors, as well as our personal, situational and systemic context at the time. A further approach to understanding the personality and what may create these patterns is to recognise that splits can occur as a consequence of traumatic experience, particularly in our childhood and early years, which result in the emergence of different parts of our personalities. This is because our personality is less a consistent harmonious unity and more a multitude of parts that are reactivated by people and situations that we meet, and, depending upon where we are on our development path, we will have differing degrees of awareness of these triggers and choice about how we react or respond. Psychosynthesis offers the systemic model of subpersonalities as a way of understanding the nature and relationship of different parts of our personality and this will be fully explored in a later chapter on coaching interventions.

Here I want to briefly touch upon a different theory of the parts of the personality – Identity-orientated Psycho-Traumatology (IoPT), developed by professor Franz Ruppert, which is explained in an excellent paper, 'What has trauma got to do with coaching? Or coaching got to do with trauma?' by Julia Vaughan Smith (2015). This model shows how splits in the personality and identity structure after a traumatic experience give rise to three parts of ourselves (*healthy, traumatised, survival*), and Vaughan Smith explores how to work with these in coaching. She explains how trauma is held in the body and points towards related developments in somatic coaching to help with this.

The key point for coaches in relationship to personal development is to learn to recognise when we are operating out of our **survival** part, when a **traumatic** part is triggered and when we are relating from our **healthy** part. More often than not, swings between inflation and deflection or an inability to stay centred and grounded can be linked with the triggering of our survival part and associated subpersonalities that may be in conflict.

Above I mentioned my over-identification with *mind* as a continuing theme in my personal development. This can also be seen as a split in my psyche in my early life, giving rise to the emergence of mind-identified survival parts (which I can associate with archetypal subpersonalities such as the critic, teacher, judge, analyst, etc.). As I started to fully recognise this survival part (and thus step outside survival and into my healthy part), I suddenly experienced a psychic release and an energetic dropping down into my being. The split between mind and heart was in some alchemical way healed at an essential level, and I have been able to draw upon this experience again when needed. I have told this story to illustrate how these different approaches to psychological health and personal development connect up, or can be seen to be tackling the same issues from different perspectives.

The wider topic of the nature and structure of mind and its relationship to consciousness and Self is important, but a step beyond the scope of this book. This includes understanding the distinction between our concrete mind, which works at the level of rationality and practicality, and our abstract mind, which opens our conceptual and imaginal capacities and builds a bridge to accessing the Self. This topic is an example of what is also best to learn about and understand experientially and interactively if we can, such as on the two- or three-year programmes run at the Institute and Trust in London. The two-year MA programme at the Institute has been re-positioned as an in-depth personal development journey in psychosynthesis. This can then be followed by clinical training to qualify as a counsellor, therapist or coach. The Trust offers a one-year foundation programme in psychosynthesis, followed by two or three programmes to qualify as a counsellor or therapist.

That concludes this somewhat extended odyssey through the territory of personal development and the models that might be useful to the coach both in working on themselves and in increasing their awareness of their coachees' issues and challenges. I have deliberately switched between speaking to our own personal development and that of our coachees, because that is how I experience needing to work on our development alongside our practice. We have touched upon some important psychosynthesis concepts alongside some of the most common psychological and personality models in use today. We have spent some time establishing the personal development context that needs to underpin our professional development as a psychosynthesis coach.

Chapter 11

Leadership development

How does psychosynthesis inform and support leadership development in coaching?

Leadership development overview

Assagioli's model of individual self-actualisation and self-realisation is our orienting model for coaching within the context of personal development, and consequently leadership development too. This model helps us hold the tension between Self (self-realisation) and Will (self-actualisation) in our curiosity about the developmental journey of our client. We explained and explored this model in Chapter 3 on the topic of personal development.

Alongside this we need to expand our perspective so as to navigate the complexities and nuances of leadership development. We therefore distinguish three distinct aspects or modes of leadership development: horizontal, vertical and inner development. The first two are widely recognised in the organisational development (OD) field, which is why I adopt this lexicon. The distinction and interplay between horizontal and vertical development is currently an increasingly popular topic within leadership development circles (see Torbert, 2014). To complement these and offer something new to the discourse amongst OD professionals, I have made the further distinction of *inner development*, which I would argue fills a gap that exists in understanding how leadership development takes place.

In simple terms, ***horizontal development*** concerns your capabilities, competencies and skills and is usually assessed using competency frameworks or aptitude-type tools. Horizontal development is essentially about how good you are at what you do or want to do and about getting better at it. Most HR departments in large organisations have their own competency models and approaches, often linked to 360 feedback and appraisal or review practices. Relevant outputs from these can be combined with leadership profiling as part of leadership development planning.

Vertical development concerns your core intelligences (primarily cognitive, but also emotional, social, ethical, spiritual, strategic, etc.), your underlying belief system and orienting perspective, your internal way of looking at and making sense of the world, as described in terms of developmental stage models (usually summarised as paradigms, worldviews or value systems), which describe the progression from relatively simple to increasingly complex and sophisticated thought systems. The Leadership Development Framework (LDF) offered by Harthill, based upon the work of Fisher and Torbert (2007), Jane Loevinger, Susanne Cook-Greuter and others is currently the most commonly used assessment tool for vertical development.

Inner development concerns deeper psychological and psycho-spiritual dimensions, such as the healthy development of our inner self, awareness and will, our core identity and personality, our desire and capacity for growth, self-realisation and self-actualisation. Inner development complements and supports both vertical and horizontal development but is not usually included explicitly within leadership development approaches. Assessment within this domain is more personal and subjective, although some tools have been developed (see below). Leadership coaches require relevant psychological training and development to be able to work with their clients at this level. Inner development is 'where the action is', as Ken Wilber once described the development of the self or the I, and can be seen as the driver, or at least the fulcrum, for vertical development and, to some extent, horizontal development.

The **inner development of leaders** can also be viewed in terms of the metaphor of alchemy. The *crucible* is the leader's sense of purpose and values, their pull towards meaning and growth, which create a context for personal development, whether conscious and articulated or not. This is the place of confrontation between the life we have so far lived and the potential of the Self and Will referred to earlier. The *elements* include the interplay of *awareness* and *will*, and the harnessing by the will of the psychological functions (such as thinking, feeling, sensing, intuition, imagination) and other resources, as well as the challenges and opportunities the leader is faced with in their work context alongside the contents and landscape of their journey. The mysterious *process* of development itself can be described in terms of the personal journey towards self-actualisation and self-realisation, or in terms of lines and levels of development (e.g. see Wilber's integral model or Frederic Laloux's leadership paradigms). Who is the *alchemist* or conductor of all this? In psychosynthesis terms we view the 'higher Self' as an inner guide. Part of the coach's role is to nurture the client's sense of *I-Self* and connection with the *higher Self*, to facilitate the process of inner development. Every client has their own inner alchemist, which we are seeking to awaken through the coaching engagement.

Five dimensions of leadership

Our core psychosynthetic model for coaching and developing leaders is Roger Evans' Five Dimensions of Leadership (5DL), and in my framework above 5DL is also our key model of inner development. The five dimensions are *'the small number of underlying human dimensions that, when developed to significant levels and come together in an individual, then remarkable and great human leadership can take place'* (Evans, 2020).

The sequence and the interrelationships between the dimensions of leadership (DLs) are important, and in his 2020 book Evans unfolds the genealogy of their emergence, drawing out their key interdependencies. Each DL is unpacked in detail, with case stories and guidelines about how to apply it to oneself or to the leaders one is coaching. Evans encourages the leader to assess themselves (and, by implication, for coaches to mentally assess the leaders they work with) in relation to each DL on a scale of 0–5. In the courses and workshops that Evans runs on 5DL for leaders and coaches, he introduces specific tools to support this. Over many years of using this model in leadership coaching, I have internalised the model and find I can mentally assess leaders quite easily and intuitively after interviews or coaching sessions. When comparing scores with colleagues, a close correspondence is generally found.

At the same time, I have noticed that my initial assessment of a leader might change as I get to know them, so it is important to always remain open, curious and inquiring when using this method.

Below are my reflections upon how each leadership DL relates to coaching:

DL1 – the ability to self-reflect is the foundation stone on which all the other DLs are built. It is therefore a key focus within leadership coaching, as we seek to support our client's capacity for self-reflection. As we have already noted, self-reflection is also our first meta-competency in the PCL coaching skills model.

Table 11.1 The Five Dimensions of Leadership defined, from *Evans (2020)*

1DL	Ability to self-reflect – self awareness
2DL	Awareness of one's impact on others, understanding difference and group dynamics
3DL	The ability to consistently see the whole picture and the dynamics between the part and the whole. The art of thinking systemically and understanding system forces
4DL	Individual freedom (free will) to both make clear decisions and then to drive delivery in the face of resistance, to be blown in the wind, to bend but to stand firm
5DL	The ability to ask for appropriate help and support – internally and externally to the organisation

In his workshops, Roger Evans offers an invaluable rule of thumb for the coach to calibrate the client's level of awareness in relationship to unhelpful, dysfunctional or unconscious blocking behaviours. Here the coach might ask the client which level of awareness they are currently capable of and then track progress over a number of sessions towards greater awareness and choice:

1.   *Don't become aware until I reflect back on what happened and then see what was going on and how caught I was, what was happening or going on with me*
2.   *Become aware of what's going on while it's happening and can't do any-thing about it; still caught but much more aware*
3.   *Aware of what is happening with me while it is happening and able to do something about it. No longer caught – much freer*

From RHE 5DL: Institute of Psychosynthesis
training material, 2018

DL2 – awareness of one's impact on others is a capacity that the coach may gradually discern from working with their client over time. However, it also points towards the need to ask for and receive feedback, either informally or formally using a 360 feedback exercise. As coaches, we are always looking for significant gaps between the leader's self-perception and the way that others see them or are impacted by them. A good place to start here is to gain the client's buy-in to running a 360 feedback exercise at the start of the coaching relationship.

DL3 – thinking systemically is increasingly critical for successful organisational leadership. It is so important that the coach is able to engage with the leader in relation to this and we focus on this in the next chapter. In simple terms, this capacity is part of what might distinguish the leader from the manager. It is also the critical capacity that is tied up in the emergence of worldviews or value systems beyond conventional *conformist* and *achievement* paradigms, as we later explore in Chapter 13.

DL4 – free will is also critical in psychosynthesis coaching when working with trifocal vision, as it is the essence of 'working in the gap'. Where there is little free will, we might need to work to identify very small steps that can help to release available will. Where there is abundant free will, we might be more challenging and supportive of our clients to encourage them to extend their reach and move beyond what they conceive is possible or comfortable.

DL5 – ability to ask for help is central to the coaching relationship. Without it, the client is unlikely to find themselves in any kind of coaching relationship. Without enough of it, the coaching may not be successful.

Development and crises of transition

All human beings develop and grow in ways that are unique and individual to themselves, while at the same time there are recognisable patterns that are common to us all. Distinguishing and exploring the modes of horizontal, vertical and inner development helps us to make sense of this highly complex topic. Some people will remain relatively stable within their vertical development for most of their adult lives, whereas others will experience continuing progression throughout their lives, or distinct periods of crisis and transition from a centre of gravity at one stage to another. We might therefore distinguish between **vertical developers** and **horizontal developers**. In broad terms, horizontal development is associated in the Assagioli model we introduced earlier with self-actualisation or personal development, and vertical development with self-realisation or transpersonal development. Horizontal developers might become very good at what they do but change little in terms of their outlook on the world. For example many successful business people are horizontal developers – Richard Branson's *Enterprising-Social*, or Alan Sugar's *Autocratic-Enterprising* styles of leadership don't appear to have changed much over their decades of business success. Obviously, some people experience both horizontal and vertical development, or go through periods of each at different times in their lives. Inner development works in conjunction with both, although an intense or tumultuous period of inner change characterised by some form of internal or external crisis is often associated with a shift between paradigms (Laloux) or value systems (Graves) as part of vertical development. An inner crisis of meaning, identity or purpose is the most obvious signifier that one is currently going through a shift or transition between paradigms or value systems.

Inner development and synthesis

Another psychosynthetic model of human development, which I believe has unrealised potential within leadership coaching, is the *triphasic model*, as developed by Joan Evans for the Institute, and drawn extensively upon psychosynthesis counselling and therapy. The model *'describes life stages through linear time, (although) it is not linear but cyclical, with each level enfolded in the other, with developmental stages resonating throughout the system'* (Evans in Simpson et al., 2013, p26). The model concerns the Self's drive towards synthesis through interdependently connected levels of pre-personal, personal and transpersonal expression, as we play out issues of separation, identification and disidentification. Figure 11.1 gives a basic representation of the model.

I anticipate that this model will help us with the next level of understanding of how inner leadership development takes place. In my own study and inquiry in this direction I am exploring how this might combine with each

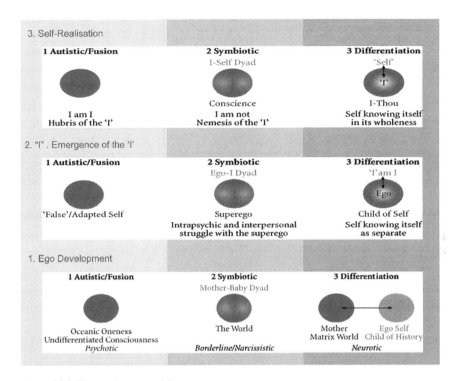

Figure 11.1 The triphasic model.

Reproduced by kind permission of The Institute of Psychosynthesis, London 2020.

of the stages of development in Laloux's or Graves' developmental systems. I will return to continue this topic at some point in the future, but will not unpack the model any further here.

Conclusion

In summary, it is important to acknowledge that leadership development is a vast and complex topic with many different perspectives and approaches. In this chapter I hope I have provided a useful framework that helps with the integration and synthesis of these different approaches. We expand upon particular aspects of leadership development in more depth in different ways in some of the subsequent chapters, for example 'vertical development' in Chapter 13. The topic as such overlaps and intersects with our central focus of explaining a psycho-spiritual approach to leadership coaching, but really needs its own space to be fully expounded upon. I plan to do this in a future book on evolutionary leadership. In particular, the full argument for inner development and its pivotal role in enabling vertical and horizontal development needs to be made.

A coaching story: *Readiness for sale*

To all outward appearances, Chris was a very successful CEO who was leading the organisation through an important period of change, as they prepared the company for sale. There was no doubt that Chris 'delivered' and had brought the organisation to the impressive place it was today. However, his way of working was very focused, constantly applying high pressure to achieve results, which often caused conflict, stress, tension and even burnout. The Chair was worried about Chris, but also worried about the impact of his style and how it was contributing to a growing sense of instability and crisis in the organisation.

Chris welcomed the idea of coaching and the 360 feedback exercise that the coach proposed they start with to give him more awareness of his wider impact. Alongside the pressures of his role, Chris's personal life was also in crisis and he realised he needed to take time out to reflect and consider who he was and where he was in his life. He also welcomed the idea of a personalised leadership development programme, given his lack of formal management or leadership training in the past.

The 360 exercise revealed both very appreciative acknowledgement of his strengths and very direct feedback about his behaviours that didn't work – which included being domineering, dismissive and blaming. It also showed the impact this was having on morale and the culture – he managed his people in silos to solve problems and drive deadlines, but there was a lack of teamwork or a sense of shared vision and purpose. Chris's tendency to idealise or scapegoat individuals within the team meant people often felt they were either in or out of favour.

He worked with the coach to look beyond the behaviours to the mindsets and patterns of thinking and personality edges that unconsciously drove them. They used profiling tools and psychological diagnostics to assist with increasing Chris's self-awareness and ownership of his behaviour. The twice-monthly sessions became an important 'time-out-of-time' for Chris, a place to reflect more deeply on his day-to-day challenges and make decisions about how he wanted to be a leader going forwards. He had listened seriously to the feedback and made a commitment to himself to be different. Immediately people started to notice this difference and, although there were occasional lapses into old patterns, he would pick himself up and recommit to the change he was making in his style of leadership.

The coach inwardly reflected about this change that was taking place for Chris and the role they could play in supporting it. The crisis in his personal life, combined with the stress he created in his work, had led to a crunch point of painful awareness and a window of opportunity had opened up. The role the coach played was mostly to listen, to witness, to challenge and support. Sometimes they would guide Chris to work on more deep-seated issues or reflect upon fundamental questions. Chris could bring the whole of himself to these sessions and this started to heal splits in his personality. The coach sought to nurture Chris's free will and capacity to make choices about how he wanted to be, by encouraging and validating each small step he made towards a new way of leading.

Each of Chris's direct reports accepted his invitation to undertake the same 360 feedback exercise along with leadership development coaching. The coach worked with the team off-site to create a shared vision and strategy, which included establishing a wider management team and starting the process of empowering and delegating responsibility to this team. Together they created the stability, succession and empowered culture needed to make the proposed sale possible and credible. The sale eventually took place and exceeded all expectations.

Chapter 12

Organisational systems and the systemic perspective

How does psychosynthesis coaching work at the organisational level? How does it engage with organisational systems? How does a systemic perspective enhance our work as leadership coaches? How do we develop the capacity for systemic awareness in the leaders we coach?

Widening the view

Since Assagioli's day, three key areas of theoretical development have emerged which I would suggest are important as to how psychosynthesis is now taken forwards, with each building upon and expanding work he had already started. These are the *systemic* perspective, the *developmental* perspective and the *somatic* perspective. There are of course overlaps between these perspectives and some of the proponents of different approaches I will touch upon might argue that their approach embraces all three of these and more.

To illustrate my point regarding these fields of latter-day development, here are some examples of key thinkers in these three areas:

Systemic: Senge, Oshry, Hellinger, Whittington
Developmental: Wilber, Graves, Wade, Kegan, Torbert, Laloux
Somatic: Strozzi-Heckler, Aquilina, van der Kolk

The developmental (or more specifically an adult-worldview-developmental) perspective is the topic of the next chapter, and the somatic perspective the chapter after that. Here we will focus on the broader systemic perspective and why it is so important to coaches working with leaders in organisations.

Language can become a barrier to understanding in this territory, so I will make some distinctions at the outset. Within the wider umbrella of the systemic perspective, I will distinguish three primary sub-topics or lines of inquiry and learning for the leadership coach.

The first is *embracing the systemic perspective* as an aspect of complexity theory and the basic implications of this. The second is *how to increase*

our understanding of human systems, in particular group and organisational systems, and how to work or intervene within them. The third
is *how to awaken or increase the capacity for systemic awareness* in the
leaders we support.

The systemic perspective as an aspect of complexity theory

In my view, over the last twenty years the most noticeable shift, across not
only the organisational world but also a wide range of professional disciplines, has been towards a growing awareness and acceptance of the systemic
perspective. Curiously, very few people (that I have noticed!) have commented
on this phenomenon and its implications, so I feel compelled to say a little
about it here.

The systemic perspective recognises the systemic nature of all aspects of
human life and affairs, from intra- and inter-personal, family and social
systems to our organisational, societal and global systems. It encompasses
systems thinking, systemic awareness and systemic practice, and has its
origins in complexity and complex adaptive systems theory. It translates
understanding of how systems work in the natural world to how systems
work in the human domain. Pretty much everywhere I go now (admittedly
in psychological, coaching and leadership circles) people talk in terms of
both the immediate human systems they are involved in as well as the wider
systems which influence these, or at least understand what I mean if I talk
about the influence and importance of these systems. This is a really massive
shift, so much so that when this kind of talk draws a 'blank look' I am quite
surprised. Twenty to thirty years ago we would speak in terms of the influence
of national and organisational culture in similar ways, but nearly all of this
talk has shifted towards the much broader and more useful systemic perspective (of which culture is still an aspect).

Arguably this shift follows the most interesting track of scientific theoretical development since Assagioli's day and has impacted almost every field of
human study and endeavour in important and different ways. Despite this,
however, there are still dead zones in terms of areas of human affairs and
problem solving which remain untouched by this essential perspective. The
whole climate change issue, for example can be viewed in terms of the degree to
which a systemic perspective is being taken in addressing the different aspects
of the problem and the solution. Tragically and laughably the academic world
(and many areas of human affairs that are over-identified with traditional
science for systemic and historical reasons, such as medicine) still seriously
lags behind in adopting systemic perspectives and adapting complex adaptive
systems theory to their respective fields. To spell this out, if it is not obvious,
most modern medical science still treats the human being as a collection of
unrelated parts rather than a whole system; individual medical interventions

are still made without considering even the most basic implications that one is treating a systemic whole human being, and many treatment approaches which draw upon systemic perspectives are considered unscientific and denied resources. Sadly and ironically in areas such as medicine, it is the shrill voice of scientific orthodoxy which is most guilty of this performative contradiction (which means asserting something which undermines the case they are asserting) through its obstinate ignorance of the greatest scientific advances of the last thirty years – in the area of complexity and systems theory. An obvious indication of the backwardness of academia is the continuing focus on very narrow conventional disciples in academic study – whereas most emerging professions and related future problem-solving demand interdisciplinary approaches.

Let me briefly illustrate some of the key principles of a systemic perspective:

1   *Systems are wholes which are more than the sum of their parts:* wholes become seen as equally important to, if not more important than, the parts. The major traps of scientific reductionism and partialism are countered or even disappeared.
2   *Systems involve a multitude of complex interrelationships and interconnections between different elements*: multiple and complex interconnections (e.g. impacts, feedback mechanisms and unintended consequences) become accepted as part of all human systems even if they are beyond our conscious awareness.
3   *Human systems are open systems which are interconnected with countless other systems*: All systems are recognised as interconnected with other systems, so we become less inclined to deal with solving problems in one system in isolation to other systems.
4   *The way human systems work includes but also goes beyond the personal and interpersonal*: disidentification increases and the emotional charge reduces as we recognise the power and influence of systems forces in our lives and affairs. We become less inclined to blame ourselves or others and more inclined to inquire about how the system works.
5   *All human systems encompass the past, present and future*: The past, present and future become seen as more linked and interconnected through the system and we start to find ways to both learn how memory of the past is held in the system and draw understanding from the past as well as to project more openly and accurately into the future.
6   *Human systems work through individual and collective consciousness and unconsciousness*: The interconnectedness of (and constant movement or energy and consciousness between) the conscious and unconscious at individual and collective levels becomes more real and apparent in ways that had not previously being recognised.

Assagioli clearly took a systemic perspective and was thinking systemically in the way he referred to organisations as living organisms, for example.

His egg diagram is a systemic perspective on how the human psyche works and his model of subpersonalities is a systems view of the personality. His understanding of the nature and process of synthesis was years ahead of its time and is still essential learning for anyone seeking to resolve complex systemic issues involving tensions between polarities. In all important ways every aspect of psychosynthesis is congruent and works in conjunction with a systemic perspective. This perspective just didn't appear in any significant way in public or academic consciousness in Assagioli's day. In his writing Assagioli frequently seeks to show how his work is consistent with scientific principle and methods – so it is a shame that he was not able to see the remarkable emergence of the systemic paradigm in the scientific world during his lifetime.

Following the work that Assagioli undertook in this area, the systemic perspective has continued to be incorporated within the world of psychosynthesis by continuing practitioners and developers. From my own direct experience this includes Roger Evans and Joan Evans, who have both made significant contributions in practice, teaching and writing. As an example, and as already mentioned above, Roger Evans' Five Dimensions of Leadership highlight the importance of systemic thinking for leadership (Evans in Simpson et al., 2013) and Joan Evans writes about her work on systems, synthesis and group dynamics (in Simpson et al., 2014).

Working with human systems in leadership coaching

Leadership coaching involves working with individuals and teams as part of an organisational system, and this brings a level of complexity and challenge for the psychosynthesis coach in at least two main ways. First of all, working with an individual leader involves holding awareness and curiosity about the organisational systems of which a client is part. Secondly, the coach can also be working at three different levels – individual, team or group and organisation or system – sometimes simultaneously. It is easy to fall into the assumption that coaching takes place only at an individual level. Leadership team coaching is becoming increasingly common and, to some extent, so is the notion that we can coach and develop organisational systems (of course, we would previously call these activities facilitation and consulting).

Working with organisational systems in coaching

Between 2003 and 2015, I worked in Roger Evans' coaching team at Creative Leadership Consultants and, as part of our supervision and reflective practice as we worked with our organisational clients, we included this basic model of three interconnected levels and thus deepened our awareness of systems forces and dynamics. This was enhanced by working with early versions of Roger's Five Dimensions of Leadership (5DL), particularly in relationship to assessing individual leaders' capacity and readiness to lead change successfully, but also as part of supporting their longer-term development. During this period, we learnt to work as a team of coaches, to see the bigger system in play and make sense of the systems forces by transcending the individual ways in which we might be caught by the system (often reflecting how our clients were caught). What are systems forces? From Joan Evans (in Simpson et al., 2014, p8):

> An organisation is a complex system which has developed over time with the individuals interacting within it. These interactions, and the impact of the culture in which it finds itself, gives the organisation an identity which includes levels of consciousness which have history, mindsets, ways of being and behaving in relationship to others both within and without the system. Going back to the initial conditions of any organisation we find that these ways of being have been set in motion quite unconsciously.
>
> Individuals can enter into the system at any point of its history and find these systems forces to which they are unwittingly subjected.

Systems thinking, and the related field of complexity or complex adaptive systems theory as applied to organisational practice (e.g. by Patricia Shaw (1997)), can be traced back to diverse origins (e.g. Ludwig von Bertalanffy's General Systems Theory (1969)) but was brought to the fore by Peter Senge who, in *The Fifth Disciple* (1990), identified the capacity to think systematically as critical for modern leadership. Barry Oshry's *Seeing Systems* (2007) provides some simple narratives, pathways and tools for helping leaders become more aware of the organisational systems of which they are part, and this is brought to life experientially in *The Organisational Workshop* which can be run for groups and teams. I have found that the simple central model of Tops, Middles, and Bottoms creates immediate recognition in most groups of what it is like to be caught in organisational systems dynamics. Recognition is needed before meaningful disidentification can take place, leading to increasing awareness and the possibility of greater freedom to act within the system. More recently, John Whittington has developed an approach to systemic coaching which builds upon the family constellations work of Bert Hellinger (1999). He identifies the hidden forces in systems to work with as *Time* (who came first in this system?), *Place* (everyone needs to find or be given a place in the organisation) and *Exchange* (has there been a fair exchange of value or energy?). He explains how the human need for belonging gives rise to powerful forces, including conscience, guilt and innocence and loyalty. He shows how conscience is held unconsciously in play at different levels in systems – for example the personal, organisational and systemic – and can be traced back to the very origins of the organisation, and sometimes beyond. As Joan Evans states, '*it is sometimes difficult to understand that the seeds for dynamics in the here-and-now have their roots in the past – and sometimes the ancient past*'. (Evans in Simpson et al., 2014, p4).

From a coaching perspective, an important starting point when taking a systemic perspective is to be able to distinguish, or at least to be curious about the distinction, between genuine client interpersonal issues and apparent interpersonal problems arising out of wider systems forces. The coach needs to wonder and be curious about whether the presenting interpersonal issues a client brings to coaching are more about the client and the relationship (*What's your part in this? What might you be projecting here?*), or an enactment of a wider systemic issue (*What's the organisational history here? What might you be playing out from the wider system?*). The next step is to be able to help clients increase their awareness of the organisational system they are part of and the systems forces at play in which they might be unconsciously caught. The third step might be to help clients learn how to start making leadership interventions at a systems level which are free of their reactions to being caught in the system. This represents very sophisticated coaching indeed and is generally only possible within longer-term coaching relationships with leaders.

In their recently published *Systemic Coaching* (2020), Peter Hawkins and Eve Turner direct our attention to the wider systemic environment of the people we are coaching and argue that coaching needs to '*deliver value to all the stakeholders of the coachee, including those they lead, colleagues, investors, customers, partners, their local community and also the wider ecology*' (Hawkins and Turner, 2020, p*i*). This wider ecological awareness is becoming increasingly recognised as essential in our connected and joined-up world and is another theme I will pick up in my next book, on evolutionary leadership.

Working with group dynamics in coaching

I also want to consider how the psychosynthesis coach works with groups or teams within organisational systems, and so turn our attention to group dynamics. Joan Evans has developed the model of group dynamics within the Institute of Psychosynthesis, drawing upon the work of Steven Kull, as well as William Schutz and his development of FIRO. The following quote comes from her introduction to this topic (Evans in Simpson et al., 2014, p13):

> Group dynamics or the interaction of individuals, impact on the system as a whole and are in fact the processes which give the momentum for it to evolve. Group work and team building are so critical because it is at the level of teams and small groups that change is determined at the global level and, as such, are the agencies for change within the larger and more complex organisation.

Evans' group dynamics model describes the evolution and the group dynamics leading towards synthesis of a system, through the interaction of two fundamental principles of order and coherence on one hand and chaos and disorder on the other.

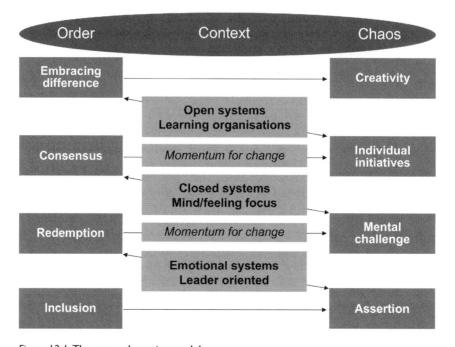

Figure 12.1 The group dynamics model.
Reproduced by kind permission of the Institute of Psychosynthesis, London, 2020.

The group dynamics model, represented graphically in Figure 12.1, '*can be applied to group work and team building as well as giving a perspective to whole systems*' (Evans in Simpson et al., 2014, p15).

How does the psychosynthesis coach work with these group dynamics? First, as a team coach they might coach team leaders so they are able to support the dynamic evolution of their team. Critically (Evans in Simpson et al., 2014, p14):

> Team leaders need to be able to sustain and face these uncomfortable dynamics since greater consciousness and higher degrees of freedom to act are the imperatives for each turn of the spiral. Thus more intelligent and psychologically mature systems come into being.

In addition, the team coach might actively intervene in the team process, during team meetings or coaching workshops. For example an external facilitator can play an important role in the inclusion process and help build trust and openness in the team. Equally, they might be able to encourage team members towards individual assertion and engage in unfiltered challenging discussion.

Secondly, as an individual coach of an individual leader, the coach can use this understanding of group dynamics to coach the leader towards building and developing their team between the coaching sessions. Most senior leaders I have coached have brought the dynamics and development of their leadership team as an issue to coaching, for which I also often draw upon Lencioni's *The Five Dysfunctions of a Team* (2002).

Incidentally, the evolutionary interplay of *order* and *chaos* (which might also be characterised in terms of structure and flow, or form and energy) in this model has similarities to Clare Graves' model of bio-psycho-social development (1970), in which the dichotomous pulls are between the *collective* and the *individual*, between human beings' needs for *belonging* and to *express* their individuality. There are also obvious similarities between the stages of group development in this model and Graves' value systems. This is not surprising, given that the same deep principles of human development are in play, whether we are looking at individual, team, organisational or societal development.

Systemic coaching and constellations

I recently spent five days training in the fundamentals of systemic coaching and constellations with John Whittington and his organisation. This is a very practical and valuable course for any coach, which both establishes a deep understanding of the principles of working with systemic constellations and provides a foundation in using a wide variety of methods with clients. This includes working in several formats: one to one, using room space or on a tabletop to map a constellation; with teams or groups in organisations to work with aspects of their systems dynamics; or with individuals on personal or organisational issues using a group of people as representatives of the elements within their system. This is powerful work which can yield extraordinary results in a very short space of time by accessing intelligence within the systemic unconscious. It combines with the somatic perspective because it involves somatic awareness: we constellate the system by asking ourselves what is our felt sense as we stand in a certain place or face in a certain direction in the constellation, or simply put a finger on an object representing something for us on a tabletop constellation of a systemic issue.

Systemic constellations work combines well with psychosynthesis coaching, and I have since developed my own approach to constellating our inner psychological space using the egg diagram and the evolutionary spiral (a topic I will visit fully in my next book on evolutionary leadership). Constellations work resonates with the group constellations and psycho-geography work we learnt on the MSc Change Agent Skills and Strategies programme in the 1990s, primarily from Paul Barber, who drew upon principles of Gestalt psychology in our work together on this.

Despite what I have written on this topic above, however, I do have some caveats and concerns about the systemic coaching and constellations approach. First and foremost, there is no clear and explicit model of the human psyche or the unconscious that underpins this practice. There is an implied philosophy or psychology, but it is not clear what that is. The theory and principles as they are concern the method and practice of facilitating constellations, not the psychology underlying this. I have observed this working well most of the time, dependent upon the skills and experience of the coach or facilitator. John Whittington himself is masterful in the way he works and provides an excellent role model for constellation facilitation. However, not everyone will be able to follow his example, especially with the practice of intuitively formulating sentences or statements to put into the mouths of representatives in a client constellation. I would be wary of advising psychosynthesis coaches to go too far in this direction, and would instead advise them to rely more upon encouraging the expression of the felt sense of the representatives and, when appropriate, to bring the client back in more actively. The other concern I have is that practitioners might end up relying too much on this single method because it feels so magical and effective in finding new answers or resolutions. Again, I would advise psychosynthesis coaches to use this approach selectively and intelligently, and to take the work forward with other coaching methods.

Increasing the capacity for systemic awareness in the leaders we coach

Finally we turn our attention to the challenge of leadership development in relationship to the systemic perspective, and wonder how we can help develop this capacity in our clients. In the next chapter I will argue that systemic awareness is the pivotal capacity in developing evolutionary leaders and we will reflect upon some broader issues in relation to this.

First of all, we should take note of the different ways of referring to this capacity by various leading thinkers. As already mentioned, Peter Senge coined the phrase 'systemic thinking' in his book *The Fifth Discipline* in 1990, but since then similar notions have been expounded in different ways, for example:

- Systems thinking – Senge
- Seeing systems – Oshry
- Integral vision – Wilber
- Systems intelligence – Hämäläinen & Saarinen *
- Integrative thinking – Martin
- Systemic constellations – Whittington
- Systems awareness (DL3) – Evans

Are all these referring to the same capacity? I would suggest that in essence they are, although different aspects and facets are emphasised each time. I would suggest there are at least three distinguishable key parts to the systemic perspective. These are:

> *Systemic awareness* – the capacity to see or sense all the systems around us and how we are caught or impacted within them, to perceive the systems dynamics and forces beyond the obvious and apparent.
>
> *Systemic thinking* – the conceptual capacity to create complex mental models and engage in the playing out of different scenarios in one's mind in ways that simulate the systems we are engaged with (I sometimes call this *systemic engagement*).
>
> *Systemic action* – the capacity to intentionally intervene or take action in relation to systems, which results in beneficial consequences.

How do we develop these capacities? How might we help develop them in others? I believe this topic warrants serious study if it has not already taken place. For now, I would like to suggest some aspects that combine to build these systemic capacities:

- Conceptual expansion – stretching the capacities of the abstract and creative mind
- Disidentification – distinguishing personal stuff from systems forces
- Emotional maturity – moving beyond being caught by ego and the parts
- Somatic awareness – inner sensory awareness-building
- Field awareness – extending our awareness outwards
- Interpersonal awareness – right relationships with others
- Group dynamics awareness – groups as organic systems
- Systemic working with constellations – with individual and group inner and outer space

There may be others and there may be important ways in which they sequence or combine to build systemic capacity. (This is a topic to be researched for my next book, on evolutionary leadership.) For now, speaking to the leadership coach, I would recommend focusing on developing systemic awareness within the coaching relationship as a first step. As part of this, it is important to encourage systemic awareness at different levels for the coachee. There are some obvious benefits from this – by shifting attention between the levels we build capacity to see all the various systems operating in the coachee's, life as well as the bigger system they are all part of. We may also come across insights at one level that help us resolve stuck-ness or over-identification at another level. We may also identify the level or levels at which the coachee is most over-identified and least able to see what is going on, and therefore needs to work on. The systems levels I am referring to are:

- *In our inner selves* – for example within the psyche at pre-personal, personal and transpersonal levels of consciousness
- *In our personal lives* – for example family systems, social systems, professional and work systems
- *In organisations* – for example teams, groups, sub-organisations, whole organisations, intra–extra systems
- *In society* – for example multiple identities, communities, regions, nations, religions, interest groups, global movements, social media

The capacity of the coach to be able to work between these levels and know when to shift attention from one to another is important. Different clients may have a clear preference to work at one level or another, and we should be curious about why this is and consider challenging them to shift their awareness. We noted in an earlier chapter how some coachees will have a bias for working on the inner world and others for the outer world. The alchemical magic of coaching often results from the continuing dialogue between the inner and outer, or between the different levels and the insights or realisations that come to the coachee when the whole system and their struggles within it come into view.

---

* Hämäläinen & Saarinen (2007) define systems intelligence in terms of intelligent behaviour within the context of complex adaptive systems: *'a subject acting with systems intelligence engages successfully and productively with the holistic feedback mechanisms of her environment. She perceives herself as part of the whole, the influence of the whole upon herself as well as her own influence upon the whole.' Observing her own interdependency with the feedback-intensive environment, she is able to act intelligently.'*

A coaching story: *Systems within systems*

Hanna was experiencing a growing dilemma with her client Rachel, who was the super-head teacher at a high-performing school. Hanna could see the systemic forces which held the current situation with all its tensions in place. She could see the forces at play in the educational system as a whole, which focused so much on targets and league tables and would celebrate head teachers who were able to turn around poorly performing schools. She could see the way that this school had become dependent upon Rachel as the dynamic leader who had turned the situation around, initially with some innovative ideas and the sheer force of her personality, and now through constant pressure on her deputies and department heads to deliver results. She could see how unhealthy ways of working and certain practices (e.g. fire-fighting by excluding difficult students) had become ingrained within the school system and were continuing unchallenged.

And now she could see how the way she worked with Rachel and her team had become part of holding this together. As their coach, she would pick up the pieces and put them back together again. She listened to Rachel's deputies in their monthly sessions, helping them develop the skills and emotional resilience to weather the storms and refocus on their goals, working too at the level of their own personal development to make meaning of the challenges they faced. She would do her best to let Rachel become aware of the impact her style was having at the same time as helping heal her own emotional wounds. Rachel would make promises to change, once this crisis, Ofsted (schools inspectorate) review or exam cycle was over. Now Alison, the key deputy who held the staff group together, had served notice to quit and Hanna could only agree that this was the right decision for her to make.

With her supervisor Hanna had acknowledged how she had got caught in this system, playing out the role of rescuer that she had learned from her own dysfunctional family of history. And she had decided she must quit too. Her supervisor asked, 'Where has this decision come from within you? As you step back from Rachel and her team, who do you see? And what are your options for how you might do this?' Hanna reflected deeply about her own process and the need to separate out from her co-dependency with the client system and its pressures of Ofsted inspections, league tables and managing the day-to-day running of the school. They worked together through different options, scenarios and strategies and arrived at a plan. They talked about the system at different levels and explored how to make interventions that could fundamentally change the systems dynamics.

At her next session with Rachel, Hanna unpacked a three-month plan for how she proposed to help the school leadership team become more resilient and able to navigate change. Rachel pleaded with Hanna to stay at first, but soon realised she was serious about leaving. She agreed to start seeing a therapist and allowed Hanna to facilitate a new contract between her and the deputies. She set about finding a replacement for Alison in a way that would involve the whole team. The deputies set up an internal coaching service for the heads of department, with external training, supervision and support. Hanna worked intensively with each of her coachees for three months towards building both greater self-sufficiency and collaborative working within the leadership team. A monthly dialogue forum was started to explore the school's culture. On the day of Hanna's last sessions with the team, they held a small party with tears, gratitude and hope for the future.

Chapter 13

The developmental perspective

How does the developmental perspective complement or augment the psycho-spiritual perspective? How might psychosynthesis be combined with developmental psychology and various approaches within this?

Why does Assagioli's psychosynthesis need updating with the developmental perspective?

This is about a very human story of the history and evolution of ideas, on the one hand, and the lives and relationships of the significant figures in this field on the other. There is a real tragedy at the centre of it, which concerns the untimely early death of Abraham Maslow at the age of 62 in 1970. Assagioli and Maslow clearly enjoyed a very creative exchange in the development of their respective works and their partnership was epitomised by the creation of the *Journal of Transpersonal Psychology* in 1969. During the same period, in the late 1960s, Maslow enjoyed an exchange of ideas with the American psychologist Clare Graves, who had originally set out to confirm Maslow's 'hierarchy of needs' model of development with his own research involving interviews with large numbers of university students. As it happened, the data led elsewhere and he ended up evolving his own *emergent cyclical levels of existence theory* (Graves, 1970). There was an ongoing exchange of ideas between Maslow and Graves (see Todorovic and Cowan, 2005), which apparently culminated in Maslow accepting the most basic difference in Graves' theory from his own – that the structure of human development and evolution was emergent, unfolding and possibly never-ending, thus turning Maslow's pyramid, culminating with self-actualisation, upside down, into an emergent cyclical spiral. Anecdote has it that Maslow was about to publish a paper acknowledging Graves' work shortly before he died. One assumes that Maslow was also unable to share his latest thinking with his friend Assagioli because of his premature demise.

The following is a short extract summarising the basic principles of Graves' model (1970, p133). I will describe the stages of development (which are mostly the same as Laloux's) in the next section:

The psychology of the adult human being is an unfolding, ever-emergent process marked by subordination of older behavior systems to newer, higher order systems. The mature person tends to change his psychology continuously as the conditions of his existence change. Each successive stage or level of existence is a state through which people may pass on the way to other states of equilibrium. When a person is centralised in one of the states of equilibrium, he has a psychology which is particular to that state. His emotions, ethics and values, biochemistry, state of neurological activation, learning systems, preference for education, management and psychotherapy are all appropriate to that state.

According to this conception we do ourselves a disservice by arguing whether man's nature is good or bad, active or reactive, mechanical or teleological. Man's nature is emergent. What man is cannot be seen before. We can see it only insofar as it has been revealed to us by his movement through the levels of human existence. And, what has been revealed to us, so far, is that in some way or another man's nature is all of these and more. Our very conception envisages that new aspects of man are now before us which were not seen before, and that man will go on proliferating into new forms if the conditions for human existence continue to improve.

Graves talked about his theory as *bio-psycho-social*, in a way that resonates with Assagioli's term *bio-psychosynthesis*. I would like to believe that this concept and model of development would have appealed to Roberto Assagioli. I don't suppose I have any way of knowing whether this was the case, as I can find no reference to Graves in Assagioli's work. I will keep researching.

I am not criticising Assagioli's work for not including a coherent and consistent model of human development along the lines of Wilber, Graves or Laloux – given more time I am sure he would have developed one! But I am suggesting that this has caused limitations in the way that psychosynthesis has developed since Assagioli's time and that this needs to be remedied when applying psychosynthesis to leadership coaching.

How does the adult-worldview-developmental perspective complement or augment Assagioli's psycho-spiritual perspective? To answer this I will start with an overview of Wilber's integral-developmental model, and then focus in on an adult-worldview-developmental perspective based upon Laloux's organisational paradigms.

Wilber's integral-developmental model

I will briefly summarise my understanding of Ken Wilber's integral or AQAL (all-quadrant all-level) model (see Figure 13.1). He distinguishes between four essential perspectives (subjective, objective, inter-subjective, inter-objective), various developmental lines (e.g. cognitive, emotional, social,

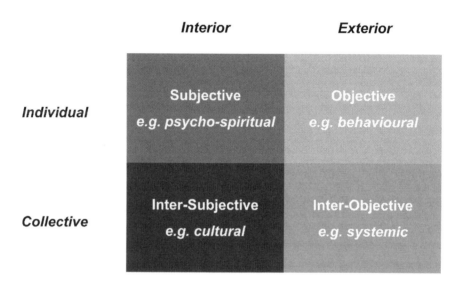

Figure 13.1 Example of Wilber's four quadrants model applied to organisational development.

strategic, spiritual, etc.), developmental stages or levels within these lines (e.g. as described by Laloux as thought paradigms – Reactive, Magic, Impulsive, Conformist, Achievement, Pluralistic and Evolutionary) and states of consciousness (e.g. sensation, emotion, concrete mind, abstract mind, intuitive mind, psychic, subtle, causal, non-dual), etc.

By 'integral', Wilber means that all the key perspectives or dimensions of human knowing are included; that we acknowledge objective as well as subjective 'truth'; that we include the exterior realm of measurable and observable behaviour as well as the interior world of values, meanings and motivations, at individual and collective levels. The above graphic is an example representation of this model, illustrating four perspectives I might typically bring to organisational development. The model can be applied to any human area of interest: to what is going on in the world; to a specific organisational situation or leadership challenge; to the fields of leadership and organisational development; to our own development as a leader, coach or other professional.

Using this framework, Wilber analyses different developmental models that have emerged over the last few decades to show how they have broad correspondence, despite arising out of different areas of focus and different research methods. He argues that they can all be accommodated alongside each other, by realising that they focus on different things or lines of development, for example Graves on value systems, Maslow on needs, Gebser on worldviews, Loevinger-Torbert-Rooke on leadership, Fowler on spirituality and so on. Within this, some models are narrower and some are broader in their focus. The *cognitive* line of development (or adult-worldview) is the broadest and most crowded in terms of different models, and Wilber tends to use this line as his way of summarising the developmental stages. In the 1990s he followed Gebser, then in the early 2000s he used Graves/spiral dynamics (e.g. see Wilber, 2000); now he seems to have switched to Frederic Laloux's model of leadership and organisational paradigms.

Wilber (1983) also developed the concept of the pre-trans fallacy, which helps enormously in contextualising and understanding the nature of human development. Below I include a brief summary of the pre-trans fallacy from an introduction to the third volume of *The Collected Works of Ken Wilber* (accessed online, 2000, np):

> The pre/trans fallacy simply says: in any recognised developmental sequence, where development proceeds from pre-x to x to trans-x, the pre states and the trans states, because they are both non-x states, tend to be confused and equated, simply because they appear, at first glance, to be so similar. Pre-rational and trans-rational are both non-rational; pre-conventional and post-conventional are both non-conventional; pre-personal and transpersonal are both non-personal, and so on. And once we confuse pre and trans, then one of two unfortunate things tend to happen: we either reduce transrational, spiritual, superconscious states to prerational, infantile, oceanic fusion (as did Freud); or we elevate infantile, childish, pre-rational states to transcendental, transrational, transpersonal glory (as the Romantics often did). We reduce trans to pre, or we elevate pre to trans. Reductionism is well-understood; elevationism was the great province of the Romantics.

The point of the pre-trans fallacy is that it helps us establish our basic orientation to development and remember which way is up. We introduce it on our leadership coaching courses at the same time as we teach the basic model of psycho-spiritual development, encompassing pre-personal, personal and transpersonal levels (as elaborated in an earlier chapter). The psychosynthetic developmental perspective is further enhanced with the triphasic model, as developed by Joan Evans (in Simpson et al., 2013) for the Institute, and which is drawn upon extensively in psychosynthesis counselling and therapy. And, as is described below, an understanding of the pre-trans fallacy and psycho-spiritual development provides valuable foundations for engaging with the adult-worldview-development perspective.

The adult-worldview-developmental perspective

The adult-worldview-developmental perspective is distinct but complementary to longer established work in developmental psychology concerning child development (e.g. Piaget, 1954) and life-stage development (e.g. Erikson, 1982). Sadly, most mainstream academic psychology teaching seems unaware of anything new in developmental psychology since Erikson's work.

The version of the adult-worldview-development perspective I have chosen to describe is that of Frederic Laloux in *Reinventing Organizations* (2014), endorsed by Wilber in the foreword. The reason for this is simple – he writes in a way that can be easily received by a broad organisational and leadership audience (unlike Wilber!) and the work is close to becoming accepted within the OD and leadership mainstream. The book caused something of a storm when it was first published (an appearance by Laloux at the RSA, hosted by Matthew Taylor, sold out) and a number of networks and websites have spun out of the evolutionary theme.

Laloux describes how his model is built upon Ken Wilber's (e.g. see *Integral Psychology*, 1999) and Jenny Wade's (e.g. see *Changes of Mind*, 1996) meta-analyses of the various models that focus on different aspects of human development (e.g. ego-identity, cognitive, moral, value systems, etc.) at individual and collective levels; these are founded on validated scientific research. The research work by Clare Graves on the emergence of value systems (probing people's conception of adult full maturity), and that of Jane Loevinger on stages of development of ego-identity, have provided the foundations for later adaptation to the organisational domain – spiral dynamics builds upon Graves' work to describe value systems in organisational terms, and the leadership development framework uses a language specific to the stages of leader development and associated crises of transition. Although their delineations of actual stages are slightly different, it is relatively easy to see how both these and other systems, derived from unrelated original research, are all describing the same *essential unfolding pattern of human development* and evolution, but from slightly different perspectives (e.g. they are looking at the same mountain from different places).

Laloux describes seven organisational paradigms that broadly follow the emergence of human consciousness and societal worldviews over thousands of years of human history, but also mirror the developmental stages that individuals follow as they grow up and mature in adulthood (at least in potentiality). These are the *reactive, magic, impulsive, conformist, achievement, pluralistic* and *evolutionary* (N.B. I will use *italics* to denote the use of these terms as names of paradigms). It may help to think of these as ways of thinking and operating in the world, which are more or less activated within an individual, group, organisation or society depending upon history, circumstance and situational factors.

Over the course of human history, we can trace the initial emergence of each new manifestation of consciousness and how the prevailing paradigm has then shifted from one to the other, but – even in today's global society – there are widely different mixes and expressions of these disparate paradigms in different societies, organisations and people. Although an individual (organisation or society) will generally have their *centre of gravity* within one or other value system, they are always expressing a unique mix of more than one, as influenced by their story and personality. In addition, everyone has the capacity for all the value systems to emerge, although the way in which this happens over time will always broadly follow the primary sequence (e.g. you can't fully activate at the *pluralistic* stage until you have in some way activated at *achievement*, and so on). Graves made a particular point that the emergence of value systems are responses to situational challenges to which the previous ways of thinking or operating are no longer providing valid or useful solutions (akin to Einstein's famous quote about problems not being solved by the same level of thinking that gave rise to them in the first place).

The transition from one paradigm to the next is often characterised by an inner or outer crisis of some kind – for example a crisis of meaning for an individual for whom the *achievement* paradigm no longer works, or the crisis of survival for an organisation which needs to outgrow a rigid *conformist* hierarchical model if it is to compete successfully with new market entrants. Turbulence, upheaval or changing circumstances have driven human progress in the past (see the work of Jared Diamond (1997) and, in the same way, it is the challenges facing today's organisations that will give rise to the new *evolutionary* paradigm emerging through new styles of leadership, cultural orientations and organisational models. At the same time, there is never a guarantee that this will happen, at least within today's organisations, and often progress follows the birth of new organisations that are more agile or adapted to present-day challenges, alongside the death of the old. Ken Wilber paraphrases Max Planck when he says '*the knowledge quest proceeds funeral by funeral*'. The history of evolution in nature is littered with long-forgotten extinct species, and human evolution with disappeared civilisations (and organisations) that failed to adapt and evolve in response to a crisis.

How the leadership paradigms evolve

I first wrote a description in 'The Influence of Leadership Paradigms and Styles on Pharmaceutical Innovation' (Howard (2016)) of how each of these paradigms emerged in human history and how they continue to emerge in human development at individual and collective levels. Below is an edited and updated version of this (which you may want to skip if you find it heavy going!).

In our description of the leadership paradigms and styles, we leave out the first worldview or paradigm, which Laloux labels *reactive*, because it is rarely found overtly in todays' organisations, although echoes of humankind's evolution as small bands surviving as foragers or hunter-gatherers between 100,000 years and 20,000 years ago are still present in our deeper psyche and collective unconscious – for example within our instincts for fight or flight in response to perceived danger. In the same way, all human beings are deeply affected and imprinted by their corresponding early experiences of dependent infancy, even though these first few months of life are beyond our conscious memory.

Magic-animistic

The *magic-animistic* leadership paradigm, which is expressed through a benevolent leadership style, is more obviously present in some form within organisations. The paradigm emerged in human history as part of the move towards tribal society some 20,000 years ago, and is often expressed and embedded through tribal or family-like metaphors or rituals within organisations or teams. It may become reactivated at times of threat to survival of the group. The organisational model and culture associated with this paradigm does not provide fertile ground for innovation or, in fact, progress of any kind at all, as the underlying thought form is one of the maintaining cycle, as in the cycle of the seasons and the performing of traditions passed on from generation to generation. The magic-animistic paradigm is most usefully found today in traditional family businesses which have remained untouched by the influence of technological progress. However, this doesn't mean that distorted expressions of associated leadership styles (e.g. patriarchal, paternalistic, materialistic) are not present in all types of organisation, usually as a consequence of psychological dysfunction on the part of individuals who unconsciously meet unresolved psychological needs by taking up permanent parental roles, beyond what is healthy in nurturing, mentoring or protecting those in their charge.

Impulsive-egocentric

In historical terms the *impulsive-egocentric* paradigm started to emerge with chiefdoms and eventually empires between 10,000 and 5,000 years ago and, in psychological terms, it represents the fully formed ego differentiating itself from parental symbiosis. It is, in this sense, the first truly individualistic (although very egocentric) worldview. The first *impulsive* organisations appeared as small conquering armies and this still represents a powerful organisational archetype today. Although street gangs and criminal organisations today can still be quite close to this model, variations can also be found in small businesses and start-ups that are driven by the energy and ego of the founder and where '*their glue is the continuous exercising of power in interpersonal relationship*' (Laloux, 2014, p18). More commonly we find both healthy and dysfunctional expressions of power-oriented autocratic styles of leadership present in all types of relationship, often masquerading as more sophisticated styles (e.g. *achievement* orientation – for good examples watch *The Apprentice* reality TV programme in the UK).

From professional observation, a generous dose of autocratic leadership style (founded on a degree of ego-narcissism, or at least an inflated sense of self-worth) is very common in a typical start-up organisation and can be seen to be part of the mix in many successful small organisations. In part, the reason may be that entrepreneurs need a degree of inflated self-belief to break through initial barriers and keep their business or project going against the odds. This can also be associated with very creative times for a business, but usually in support of the original business idea, innovation or purpose. Typically, such organisations arrive at a creative or innovative impasse at some point in their growth, unless the power-oriented leader is able to adapt his or her style or has the wisdom to allow a succession of leadership to take place. This is the first crisis of organisational growth (see Greiner, 1998 for a different perspective on this). Often this takes place by default at the point when business founders sell to a larger company or seek some kind of institutional investment. At this point, whether willingly or not, the style of leadership changes and the organisational structure formalises and develops to distribute responsibility away from the power leaders and towards smaller units. Sometimes this transition proceeds to a more formal organisational model, either inadvertently killing off the original creative culture (with people leaving) or leading to conflict between the start-up founders and the new parent leadership.

Conformist-absolutist

Here we are describing the organisational transition from *impulsive-egocentric* to *conformist-absolutist*. The historical emergence of the *conformist* mode started about 4,000 years ago, with the transition from chiefdoms to nation states and stable civilisations, and the subsequent founding of the world's great religious traditions. This has been the prevailing organisational model ever since, until the last century or two, and is still the backbone for much of what we would consider to be the establishment today – church, armed forces, government and universities for example. The conformist-absolutist organisational model is a significant progression from what came before in that *'organisations can now plan for the medium and long term and they can create structures that are stable and can scale'* (Laloux, p20). In order to grow, many organisations draw upon the conformist-absolutist paradigm by establishing clear roles, responsibilities and processes that enable this scaling. The build-up of bureaucracy, inertia and conformity that characterises this model as organisations become larger and larger (sometimes not through organic growth but by acquisition) can then become the problem. Again, this paradigm contains within it the seeds of its own destruction, or at least the death of organisations that fail to evolve beyond it in response to environmental change.

The accompanying change in leadership style is startling in its reversal away from autocratic self-orientation and opportunism – towards duty, responsibility and professional dedication. The Leadership Development Framework developed by Rooke and Torbert (2001, 2005) delineates two distinct leadership styles associated with this paradigm – the dutiful Diplomat, who conforms to and enforces the expected norm, and the professional Expert, who is dedicated to excellence within their discipline and leads as a role model for those starting out in their profession.

Achievement-multiplistic

The prevailing organisational and leadership paradigm in contemporary western society, and certainly in business organisations, is *achievement-multiplistic*. In historical terms, this form emerged in the shape of the western enlightenment movement something over three hundred years ago, and has driven not just the explosion of scientific and technological discovery, the industrial revolution and economic growth, but also the growth and dominance of prosperous, modern democratic societies. Three big breakthroughs accompany the emergence of this paradigm and inform the *enterprising* style of leadership: innovation, accountability and meritocracy (Laloux, p26). In terms that we understand today, innovation really gets going with this paradigm and leadership style. Leaders operating from this paradigm can 'live in the world of possibilities, of what is not yet but could be one day' (ibid.). There is no longer just one right way to do things but a multiplicity of possibilities. They challenge the status quo, always looking for better ways to do something, and they are open to change, uncertainly and opportunity. Thus they challenge the morbidity and hierarchical inflexibility of conformist-absolutist organisations and have invented departments that did not previously exist, including R&D, marketing and product development, as well as the project-driven way of working that has superseded the purely process-driven operating model of conformist organisations. Most of what is considered to be good leadership today is an expression of this paradigm and way of thinking – the achiever leader encourages and enables teamwork, rewards and recognises performance and leads by example.

The achievement paradigm contains within itself the seeds of new problems and is itself now the barrier to the emergence of the next leadership paradigm. This is because it mitigates against a more multi-dimensional perspective of leadership becoming widespread (it doesn't see the point, because it is confident in its own superiority as a way of looking at the world). So the achievement worldview and style of leadership has become part of the problem: by over-obsessing with the need for success in the short term (which feeds and is driven by the investment world); by focusing on success and winning rather than purpose; by over-emphasising the rational or cognitive in relationship to the emotional, social, spiritual and ethical dimensions of human beings; by maintaining the underlying limitations of the hierarchical system (as a hangover from the previous conformist paradigm) and over-focusing on management – adding more and more layers of management as the answer to most problems, rather than stripping them away to release the creativity of those who are managed. There are interesting echoes here of the fault lines in our wider modern market-capitalist society, which have become increasingly apparent since the start of the global economic crisis in 2008. We are facing crises throughout business and society, from how to deliver better health services to how to respond to climate change and, increasingly, people are beginning to realise that the answers to these crises may not come from the achievement-paradigm type of thinking.

If you are following this narrative for the first time, you might now be asking if there is a leadership paradigm representing a new shift in societal consciousness that addresses these issues of the prevailing achievement paradigm. Yes there is, but before this arrives, there has been something of a diversion (albeit an essential and valuable one) – with the rapid emergence of the *pluralistic* paradigm.

Pluralistic-relativistic

The emergence of new paradigms is seemingly speeding up as part of the evolution of human consciousness, society and culture. In the last fifty years or so, the *pluralistic* worldview has developed at an astonishing pace and now pervades many spheres of society (e.g. the arts, academia, not-for-profit organisations, left-wing politics, etc). This is the emergence of post-modernism, partly in reaction to materialistic modernism; of championing the people principle as a counterbalance to the profit principle; of the human per-spective as antidote to the mechanistic clunk-and-grind economic progress of the achievement paradigm. The *pluralistic-relativistic* paradigm brought three significant breakthroughs within organisations (Laloux page 32): empower-ment; values-driven culture; and the stakeholder perspective. These developments are now embedded in most modern large organisations, along-side (but not instead of) achievement-multiplistic principles of innovation, accountability and meritocracy. The paradigm is expressed through a more democratic, social, relational and humanistic style of leadership. People are increasingly nurtured, developed, consulted and coached by leaders. This has certainly made organisations more human places to work and has improved the experience of work for many people.

There is one problem – although there are examples of values-driven businesses delivering improved shareholder value, there are also examples where this is not the case, and even some cases where the pluralistic para-digm and associated leadership style has become too dominant and per-formance has worsened, threatening the survival of the organisation (e.g. Prudential in the early 2000s). This has contributed to distrust between achievement-multiplistic and pluralistic-relativistic leaders, to a clash of value systems between profit and people orientations, rumbling away beneath the surface. The deeper problem is that, despite the human tone that the pluralistic leadership style brings (listening, empowerment, engagement, 360 feedback, etc.), people still do not trust their organisations and will not bring their whole selves (and therefore their full creativity and innovative edge) to their work. The fact that they need to be empowered by leaders, engaged by the organisation and enrolled in its purpose, means by definition that at some point they have become disempowered (through the concentration of power at the top of organisations), disengaged and alienated from a purpose that they were not involved in coming up with in the first place.

Yet again, part of the problem is that the adherents of the pluralistic paradigm and style of leadership do not see the whole picture and set themselves against the excesses of the previous materialistic worldview. On one level, they maintain that no one's viewpoint is more valid than anyone else's, and on another they also secretly believe that theirs is the right one. Importantly, however, despite its inherent contradictions, by bringing the human being and our emotions back into the picture, the relativistic perspective lays the ground for the emergence of a truly transformative worldview, and evidence that this is finding its way into organisational and leadership expression has started to appear.

Evolutionary-systemic

Management writers, gurus and consultants have been proclaiming the next great leadership paradigm for some time and largely been missing the target (typically by oversimplifying and conflating the old paradigms and by over-idealising or over-identifying with the new one). What makes Laloux's work (2014) ground-breaking is that he has carried out detailed research concerning a dozen large organisations where the new worldview has taken shape, and describes the *evolutionary* paradigm and associated leadership styles based upon evidence of what he found in common. Importantly, he properly draws out the sequence of previous paradigms and shows how each new way of thinking and operating is both built on the gains of the previous one and is also an emergent response to its inherent limitations. He shows how evolutionary organisations can work radically differently (at once they are more effective, innovative, ecological and human to work in) from the great majority that we know and experience today. Drawing from evidence, he identities three common characteristics or principles of evolutionary organisations – self-management, wholeness and evolutionary purpose. He plays with the metaphor of organisations as living systems or organisms with a purpose of their own, in contrast to the clunky and alienating machine metaphor that identifies the achievement paradigm or the social and family metaphors that signal the pluralistic.

Laloux explores how the structures, practices, leadership styles and cultures within evolutionary organisations reflect the principles of self-management, wholeness and evolutionary purpose. He identifies the two necessary conditions for the emergence of evolutionary organisations: a sufficient level of psychological development of the top leadership (e.g. CEO or founders); and 'enlightened' owners who are willing to embrace and trust the evolutionary worldview of their leaders.

Evolutionary leaders

As leadership coaches we are more concerned with how the evolutionary paradigm emerges within leaders than how it is manifest in new organisational models, as Laloux is in his book. In practice we are likely to be coaching leaders who are working in organisations that are at all stages of development (or more likely in complex mixes of several of them) and only a very few might have an opportunity to create or nurture an organisation which embodies the evolutionary paradigm. Yet, in my experience, there is usually a desperate need for evolutionary leadership within all these organisations too. I will say more about this below, but for now I want to focus on the significance of the awakening of the evolutionary paradigm within an individual.

The shift to an *evolutionary* worldview within a leader is of a magnitude greater than any of the previous paradigm shifts. It is variously called second-tier, higher-order or meta-something for this reason. From this perspective, the leader can work with the whole system of all the previous paradigms or worldviews and see the part they play in the evolutionary process. It is not just another worldview or paradigm, but one that can work with the health of the whole system of paradigms. More importantly for this topic, research (e.g. Torbert, 2005) has shown that *evolutionary* leaders are by far the most successful at implementing large-scale corporate transformation programmes. Clare Graves describes similar findings related to creative solutions when comparing groups of people operating from different paradigms and when given complex tasks to perform. He found that the *evolutionary* group would find 'unbelievably more solutions than all the other groups put together', and of 'an amazingly better quality'. Laloux's research comes to very similar conclusions – organisations with *evolutionary* leaders are far more effective and innovative than similar organisations working under *achievement* or *pluralistic* leaders.

The Laloux system we have described culminates with the *evolutionary* paradigm. To some extent this conflates two distinct stages within Clare Graves' schema (GT/Integrative and HU/Holistic) and two stages within Torbert and Rooke's (2005) leadership development framework (*Strategist*, *Alchemist*). This is not a great problem when talking about organisational paradigms as transformational and radically different ways to look at organisations. However, when applied to leadership styles, I will maintain that it's important to make the distinction between GT/Integrative and HU/ Holistic, using the Graves model. For example the *integrative* stage is more individualistic and the *holistic* stage more collectivist in orientation. I strongly recommend not losing sight of Graves' cycling between individual and collective orientations in the developmental spiral as it helps create awareness of this tension between polarities. In my practice of profiling leaders, I have noticed quite distinct differences between these perspectives and expressions; that the *integrative* value system invariably comes first, and that little of the *holistic* value system is found in large modern organisations. Therefore, in the profiling tool that I have developed I make this sub-distinction within the *evolutionary* paradigm between *evolutionary-integrative* and *evolutionary-holistic* leadership styles.

Working with the developmental perspective – finding solutions to complex problems

Why is an understanding of this developmental system so important for leadership coaching? Firstly, this developmental approach is needed from a systemic perspective by leaders and leadership to help with the diagnosis and solution of complex systemic problems, whether societal or organisational. All complex human systemic problems have a developmental aspect which, if not seen and understood sufficiently, can lead to failure in any attempt to resolve them. This has two parts to it. First of all, the leader needs to be sufficiently activated at the *evolutionary* paradigm in order to be able to see and work with the developmental system and all the paradigms in play, without reaction or over-identification, as outlined in the previous chapter. Secondly, appropriate responses and interventions are needed to address issues for different parts of the systems which are centred in different paradigms. So, for example *conformist* elements generally need to be addressed by carefully considered *conformist-achievement* strategies. Equally, it is unlikely to work to address *impulsive* elements in the system with *achievement-* or *pluralistic*-level solutions. Many of the world's current problems have been caused or made worse by responses from a mismatched paradigm. For obvious examples of this witness the catastrophes of Iraq or Syria and the failure of modern *achievement*-level strategies to deal with *impulsive-conformist* regimes, or the widespread inability of *pluralistic* liberal politicians to respond effectively to the re-emergence of *impulsive* autocratic populists. For examples of relative success, see the Good Friday agreement in Northern Ireland or Mandela's transition to power in South Africa.

The key point is that it is not enough to simply characterise the developmental dynamics of any situation in terms of an old (bad) paradigm and a new (good) paradigm, as in much writing on change and transformation. Unless leaders engage with the systems dynamics at a sufficiently granular level and understand what specific barriers to progress are in place and how to address them, they risk provoking reaction and regression (witness Brexit, the election of Trump and other regressive shifts in recent world events). It will take a much longer book to fully elaborate these principles with guidelines and examples, but hopefully the basic principle is clear.

The above can be summarised with three key ways we work with this developmental system as coaches, which we can also support in the leaders whom we are coaching:

- Recognising the paradigms in play
- Engaging with each one effectively at its own level
- Diagnosing organisational dynamics and creating systemic solutions

How else can we work with this developmental system in psychosynthesis leadership coaching? In what other ways do we use this understanding?

- Profiling leaders in their development to increase awareness
- Matching coaches with leaders in support of their development
- Facilitating crises of transition between stages

Leadership styles awareness and profiling

I recently developed an approach to profiling leadership styles that builds upon Laloux's model of organisational paradigms, combined with useful aspects of Clare Graves' developmental model (1970), popularised as spiral dynamics. I am in the process of developing a set of tools involving self and peer feedback which can help leaders use this approach to support their leadership development.

To set the context for this, it helps to consider the dynamic between inner and outer aspects of leadership. This approach holds that a leader's inner orientation, which is made up of *constellations* of beliefs, assumptions, motivations, mindsets and ways of thinking which we refer to as *paradigms* or *worldviews*, will broadly determine or give rise to their outer expression of leadership style – although the way in which this happens on an individual basis will be influenced by the leader's unique personality, preferences, skills, experience and so on. If we were to ask a broad mix of people working in organisations what leadership style means to them, they would probably refer to styles in terms that describe their outer impact and way of operating: for example charismatic, collaborative, consensual, controlling, democratic, domineering, egotistic, empowering, encouraging, hierarchical, motivating, paternalistic, top-down, and so on.

The developmental system we are working with provides a way to see the pattern behind these different outer styles and realise that there is a progression from less sophisticated to more sophisticated styles, from styles suited to simple organisational systems and challenges to those needed to deal with the complexities of today. According to the Gravesian model (1974), alongside this progression to greater complexity there is also a cycling between individualistic value systems and collectivistic value systems – in other words, from those that emphasise individual values to those that place greater value on teams, the whole organisation and even the wider knowledge community. At each turn of the cycle, the collective orientation is always enlarging, i.e. from tribe or group to organisation or nation, and on to society or humankind.

The table below provides a quick summary of the characteristics of each paradigm and how they translate into corresponding leadership styles. Again, we are skimming the surface here and for a fuller treatment I recommend reading the first part of Frederic Laloux's book or dipping into Ken Wilber's comparative analysis (e.g. *A Theory of Everything* (2000)).

Within each stage there can be healthy and less-than-healthy expressions of leadership style, depending upon both the individual's level of psychological health and personal development and the suitability of the leadership style to the organisational situation and challenges. It has been successfully argued (e.g. by Manfred Kets de Vries, 2006, p24) that in today's modern organisational environments (centred in the *achievement* paradigm but with elements of *impulsive, conformist* and *pluralistic* modes, according to historical, market and situational influences), the people who rise to the top of hierarchical and competitive organisations are more likely to have some kind of personality pathology, and certainly to be more self-oriented, egotistic or narcissistic, than the average person. Business folklore is littered with stories of charismatic, powerful business people who, at least on the surface, have been highly successful, but around whom there has been much collateral damage in human terms. Only as the *pluralistic* paradigm starts to become stronger in an organisation is it more likely that genuinely empathetic, other-oriented, well-balanced personality types are likely to become successful managers and leaders.

The following table elaborates the leadership styles further, as recognisable leadership archetypes within today's organisations:

The evolutionary paradigm as a place to come from rather than a place to get to

Like many of my colleagues I was very excited to read Laloux's book when it was first published. I am still excited by the book and recommend it to anyone who I think might appreciate it. However, I have noticed within the movements and initiatives (e.g. websites, networks) that have grown to take the work out into the world, an emphasis whereby an opportunity is being missed, or even a wrong turn taken. I have already noted above that *in coaching* we are more interested in evolutionary *leadership* than in evolutionary *organisations* – that is, with the awakening of this paradigm within leaders as a way of seeing and engaging with the world, rather than as an organisational model to follow,

Table 13.1 Leadership styles (Howard), leadership paradigms (Laloux) and value systems (Graves) aligned

Leadership style (outer impact) and other expressions	Leadership paradigm (inner orientation) + Graves thinking mode	Cultural orientation + Organisational model + Primary motivations	Individual or collective orientation and locus of attention
Benevolent +	Magic +	Family + Circle	Collective – tribe, family or group safety
Matriarchal/Protective	Animistic (BO) Impulsive +	+ Belonging/Continuity	
Autocratic +		Power + Autocracy	Individual – own needs and wants
Egotistic/Patriarchal	Egocentric (CP) Conformist +	+ Rewards/Respect	
Hierarchical +		Role + Hierarchy	Collective – roles and rules within structures
Controlling/Systematic	Absolutist (DQ) Achievement +	+ Responsibility/Duty	
Enterprising +		Achievement + Adapted hierarchy	Individual – own and team performance
Rational/Competitive	Multiplistic (ER) Pluralistic +	+ Success/Winning	
Social +		Relationship + Flatter hierarchy	Collective – team and organisational culture
Democratic/Communal	Relativistic (FS) Evolutionary +	+ Participation/Self-expression	
Integrative +		Evolutionary + Self-management	Individual – professional networks and wider connections
Systemic/Evolutionary	Systemic (GT) Evolutionary +	+ Learning/Freedom	
Holistic +		Evolutionary + Self-management	Collective – global communities and meta networks
Transformational/Evolutionary	Holistic (HU)	+ Transformation/Purpose	

Table 13.2 Descriptions of leadership styles (based upon Laloux's paradigms)

Benevolent (*magic*) – they lead as the elder or guardian of a community. They tell stories, maintain traditions and seek to preserve the wisdom of the past.

Autocratic (*impulsive*) – they lead decisively and from the front; they are in charge. They control power and reward loyalty. Their way is the right way.

Hierarchical (*conformist*) – they lead by passing judgement according to a system of well-defined roles and responsibilities. They follow the established right way to do things.

Enterprising (*achievement*) – they lead by example and by creating opportunities for the team to succeed. They are driven to achieve goals. They constantly look for better ways to do things.

Social (*pluralistic*) – They lead by building consensus and providing opportunities for people to grow and develop. They know there is no universally right way to do things.

Integrative (*evolutionary*) – They lead by responding to situations in whatever style is needed, seeking to create synergy within the wider system. The right way is the way that works.

Holistic (*evolutionary*) – They lead by guiding others to be leaders and by creating the context for growth within a healthy system. They are constantly evolving a new way or path.

through implementing key principles. Within this context, 'evolutionary' is a place to come *from*, rather than a place to get *to* – it is a way of systemically engaging with all the paradigms in play in an organisation or social system and seeking ways to optimise the healthy functioning of the spiral, rather than another paradigm that we seek to evolve to or arrive at which is better than all the previous paradigms. This was the trap of *pluralistic-relativism*, which became another paradigm set up in conflict with the previous *achievement-materialist* paradigm. I see signs of the same happening with the evolutionary paradigm – 'once we all get to evolutionary it will all be OK!' – and I want to sound a warning.

Graves made the point that people who tested at second tier/GT/systemic in his developmental system tended to be outwardly like nothing in particular – or in other words, were adaptive in a chameleon-like way to the environment and the needs of the situation. They might appear aloof or remote at times and at other times engaged and charismatic. Other descriptions emphasise these people's lack of ego or, in our psychosynthetic terms, ability to disidentify and transcend the limitations and contents of personality. The other point is that the *evolutionary* paradigm (GU and HT in Gravesian terms) is not the end of the journey, and each paradigm will eventually become superseded by another as its limitations are exposed by an emergent crisis.

I have stuck with Graves' system as my primary map of this territory (sometimes augmenting this with the leadership language of the Leadership Development Framework developed by Torbert, Fisher and others), because of the dynamic elegance of the system as a whole – spiralling between dichotomous tensions that reflect the more universal evolutionary principle. Sometimes I find it helps to deepen understanding of this developmental system (whether focused upon individual, group, organisation or society) by drawing out the universal evolutionary shapes, principles and patterns which underlie all these levels (I ran a four-morning seminar that included this at the EFPP summer school in Doorn, in the Netherlands, in August 2019). Although tempted to include a brief version of this here, I have concluded that this should wait to be more fully explained in a future book.

A coaching story: *Wake up*

Ed's leadership styles profile had given him a bit of a shock. He knew that he was individualist in his nature but hadn't realised quite how much this was the case, with *achievement/enterprising* his standout style at 47 per cent, and 75 per cent of his profile on the side of *individual expression* (as opposed to a *collective belonging* orientation). As the recently appointed chairperson, he wanted to be seen as more team-oriented. He was also surprised to see *impulsive/autocratic* as his next most prevalent style, which he knew was an outmoded way to lead these days.

'I'm disappointed not to have a higher score for *integrative*; I thought I was further up the evolutionary ladder,' he tells the coach.

'Which part of you wants to be further up the ladder?'

'Ah, that would be my "achiever"!' laughs Ed.

'Yes, it's the same part that wants to succeed in business and helped get you here today'.

'OK, I can see that but I don't see myself as Autocratic,' Ed tells the coach. 'How does that show up?'

'Well, you could look at some of your Belbin feedback descriptors that occurred most frequently. Alongside challenging, competitive and enterprising you also have impatient, confrontational, hard driving…'

'Yes, I suppose those are fair enough and I can see why "shaper" is my highest preference in my Belbin profile. I notice I react a lot to people in meetings when they don't respond to a shortfall in the results. But if I wasn't like that nothing would get done … At the same time, I can't go on like this, I feel like it just creates too much stress'.

The coach made a note of an important mindset that they could work on in the future but then asked a different question. 'How might you be different in those meetings?'

'I suppose I could hold onto my reactions and allow time for others in the leadership team to respond'.

'Good. How else might you be different?'

'I could give Karen an opportunity to say more. She has the pluralistic/social leadership style which I seem to be missing – and the highest Teamworker preference in our group, so I need her voice'.

'That sounds important. How else?'

'By not reacting or focusing solely on targets, I might encourage people to say more about what is going on in the business. I need to start listening in a different way'.

'Ah! There I'm hearing the Integrative leader in you'.

Chapter 14

The somatic perspective

How might psychosynthesis be combined with somatic work and various approaches within this?

Somatic perspectives

As I have already highlighted, the third key area of theoretical and practical development that has been undertaken since Assagioli's day is the field of somatic work. This has many loosely associated branches, for example somatic coaching, body work, biofeedback, bioenergetics, etc. This is not a field in which I am well read or trained, and yet I sense that it also has great relevance in addressing the leadership crisis. Somehow, we need to bring the body (as well as the spirit and soul) back into organisations and find a new kind of embodied leadership that is capable of responding to the emergent crises in society.

I know that the Institute of Psychosynthesis has explored ways of bringing somatic work into counselling and psychotherapeutic practice and I have written about somatic coaching in a recent blog post (Howard, 2017c), touching on how it is important to psychosynthesis coaching.

My primary reference on this subject is a very readable book on *The Art of Somatic Coaching* (2014) by Richard Strozzi-Heckler. He sets out the central premise of somatic work, that '...*while psychotherapy focused on reasons why something is the way it is, I would ask how is it that we have formed ourselves. For example, how do we form ourselves toward contact or away from contact, instead of why don't we make contact?*' In this seminal work, Strozzi-Heckler issues a call to those interested in personal and societal evolution to wake up. He sets his somatic approach within historical, coaching and personal contexts and makes some basic distinctions between the entry points of working on, with and through the body. The book goes on to describe a methodology for somatic coaching and the importance of attending to our rhythm of energy, and ends by mapping out the somatic arc of transformation.

In *Embodying Authenticity* (2016), Eunice Aquilina (a student of Strozzi-Heckler) adds depth and breadth to the somatic narrative in a very personal and practical account that is richly illustrated with stories of how she works with leaders and organisations. She also goes some way to weaving the somatic perspective together with other important perspectives informing leadership and coaching, such as the *developmental* prism (e.g. Laloux, Kegan, Cook-Greuter and Torbert), *complexity* theory and *systemic* practice (e.g. Critchley, Wheatley, Stacey and Shaw), amongst others. Again, this shows how the three perspectives – systemic, development and somatic – weave together and work together.

Aquilina (2016, p9) speaks of the need for '*wise and conscious leaders and practitioners, who are able to tune into themselves and simultaneously tune into what is emerging in the field, taking action from a deeper sense of awareness*', and views organisations as living systems where '*leaders can bring their whole selves as fully rounded human beings and invite others to do the same… this is the offer of somatics*'.

I find Aquilina's words a profoundly resonant response to the leadership crisis within the being space. This is also very much the territory of engaging with Laloux's principle of wholeness in evolutionary organisations. She challenges the reader to engage in an inquiry into how their '*history literally shapes what has become habitual ways of being*' (Aquilina, 2016, p13). She shows how to work with the somatic arc of transformation to '*shape a new way of being in the world*'. She explores how we can use the 'self as instrument' of change, and how *through the quality of our presence, we create a strong container for others where we cultivate trust and listen beyond words…*' (ibid.).

Drawing upon Strozzi-Heckler's and Aquilina's work, below is my summary of the key principles of somatic coaching:

- Entry points for somatic practice
  - Working *on* the body – addressing presenting symptoms physically or by touch, usually by someone trained in a relevant professional modality, for example massage, reiki, kinesiology, craniosacral therapy, osteopathy, physiotherapy, etc.
  - Working *with* the body – to release blocks by working physically, energetically, emotionally, relationally, etc.
  - Working *through* the body – engaging life energy by attending to what is, what has been, what is emergent and the call of the Self

- Methodology of somatic practice
  - **Somatic awareness** – becoming aware of our sensations, to feel, to notice
  - **Somatic opening** – opening of the soma so change can occur; undoing the habitual shape to allow another shape to come to life

- **Somatic practices** – for example breath, movement, visualisation; enabling us to embody new skills and ways of being to support our goals and our emergent self

- Rhythm of energy (with the Gestalt cycle-of-experience equivalent)

  - **Awakening** – *sensation and awareness*
  - **Increasing** – *mobilisation of energy and action*
  - **Containing** – *contact and resolution*
  - **Completing** – *withdrawal and completion*

- Somatic arc of transformation (and related psychological orientations)

  - **Historical shape** – the pre-personal and the past
  - **Unbounded shape** – the personal and the present
  - **New shape** – the transpersonal and the emergent future

Some somatic coaching questions I use:

- *What is going on for you now? What sensations or feelings in your body?*
- *What's that feeling? Where do you feel that in your body? Maybe place your hand there.*
- *Do you notice your posture (or shape) as you say that? What might your posture be saying?*
- *Can you breathe into that place – what is that like?*
- *Would it help to take a deep breath? – Maybe take a few, slow deep breaths (and breathe with them).*
- *As you step into that space or place, what do you want to say? What is your felt sense?*
- *As you step out of that space or place, what do you notice or become aware of?*

Somatic psychosynthesis

This somatic approach refers to the Self as the source of our energy, wisdom and insight, and in many ways this is entirely congruent with psychosynthesis. However, in my view, in order for this work to be useful to coaches it needs to be underpinned by drawing upon a robust **psychology of self and will** (such as psychosynthesis), and a therapeutic awareness of how the different parts of ourselves come into play, such as is discussed in Julia Vaughan Smith's 2015 APECS paper and explored on her retreats. If not, the somatic practitioner is in danger of waking up parts, or releasing energies within their clients, that they are unable to deal with. We are noticing coaches coming towards psychosynthesis coaching because they are finding clients opening up to them and engaging at an emotional level that they feel ill-equipped to work with. They are looking for a stronger context for working at greater depth and height without necessarily becoming a therapist.

Just as it has become less taboo to refer to and work with *feelings* in organisations (thanks in part to the popularisation of emotional intelligence/ EQ), so too with the *body,* and it now feels much easier to refer to the body within the coaching context than it was say twenty years ago. Somatic working doesn't necessarily involve touch, and you will probably stay away from direct physical contact unless you are explicitly combining coaching with some other touch-based modality. Somatic working can involve engaging with *human form and energy* in a host of ways, including posture, shape, pattern, flow, space, rhythm, movement, stillness and breath.

I must emphasise that I have not been specifically trained in the somatic approach; however, I find it both immediately relevant and intuitively accessible as another dimension to the way that I work, whether as coach, facilitator or educator. There is a natural fit within the context of psychosynthesis psychology and the model of body–feelings–mind. Roberto Assagioli explored the deeper processes of involution and evolution and emphasised the need for human beings to work towards full embodiment as well as self-realisation – in other words, noting that we need to both come more into our bodies, anchoring in the physical plane and connected to the earth, and discover our higher nature and transcend our material fixations. Embodiment, incarnation (e.g. the journey from spirit to matter) and becoming grounded doesn't end with being born and is something we might work on our whole lives, as part of coming more into our being and presence (as I described in my story at the beginning) – in other words, connecting down as well as up – and somatic working really helps with this. I suspect this is particularly important in modern western society where cultural splits between mind and body have become endemic and where many of us are overly mind-identified (thinking is all). This may all sound a bit esoteric but, increasingly in my coaching practice, I am hearing people seeking a connection here: *I want to be more grounded and fully present… I just need space to breathe… this may sound crazy, but I feel like I'm still working towards becoming embodied…*

There seems to be a paradox at the heart of this somatic path, which is contained within the dual meaning of 'somatic': the term sometimes means *of the body*, but also more essentially means *of the body-mind* (as an indivisible whole). Much of the practice involves working through, with or on the body as the entry point, but staying mindful that in doing this we are engaging with the whole human being, mind–body–feelings, and activating all levels of consciousness.

As an example of how somatic practice works, two APECS colleagues, Fiona Adamson and Elspeth Campbell, ran a short session to demonstrate somatic coaching at the 2017 APECS Symposium. They described their session in these terms:

> Coaching-with-the-body, our felt sense of awareness, is becoming increasingly accepted as part of coaching practice. Instead of asking why

something is the way it is, we explore how it is that our sensory perceptions and emotional responses have contributed to patterns of behaviour in interactions and formed ways of being.

There is another very significant way in which the somatic perspective has informed a change in the way I work as a coach, which concerns how I approach *mindset change*, at both the individual and organisational level. We will touch upon this in the next chapter.

Somatic work and trauma

On a recent coaching course workshop, one of our students shared, with surprise, their realisation that they had been engaging in personal development for many years through the lens or filter of their **survival** self, rather than their **healthy** or authentic **self**. At the time, I thought this was an interesting observation and left it at that. At some point the next day, my unconscious having worked busily away, something troubling dawned upon me – that I had been doing exactly the same, for nearly forty years. In my case, my survival self is my mind orientation and the way I seek external acknowledgement and internal control through understanding and intellectualisation. That's not to say that I haven't experienced much of my lifetime of personal development authentically, but that my pattern is to split and intellectualise. On realising this, I experienced a profound shift, which felt like a descent into my body from my head, or into my being from my mind, and for the rest of the weekend I experienced resting in this new way of being. I felt grounded and present, at the same time able to access and engage my mind, but without detaching from my emotions or felt sense. I found it helped to place my hands on my chest or stomach, and to acknowledge my felt senses in other ways, when later sharing this experience with the group.

In the above story, I am referencing a model of the personality set out by Franz Ruppert, which is explained in a really excellent paper, 'What has trauma got to do with coaching? Or coaching got to do with trauma?' by Julia Vaughan Smith. I first saw this work published as an APECS symposium paper (2015) but you can also find it on her website. The model shows how splits in the personality and identity structure after a traumatic experience give rise to three parts of ourselves (healthy, traumatised, survival), and Vaughan Smith explores how to work with these in coaching.

She explains how trauma is held in the body and points towards related developments in somatic coaching. She concludes (Vaughan Smith, 2015, p10):

> it is my view that coaches with understanding and experience of this field (personality and self) can bring something additional to the coaching work, a greater transitional space between the inner and outer worlds,

which allows for deep transformation without working directly with the traumatised self or with the past. It needs a slightly different tool kit.

(p10)

Vaughan Smith here is answering better than I have seen anywhere else the question about the boundary between coaching and therapy, and also describing the work that we do on our psychosynthesis coaching courses very well. She has expanded her treatment of this important topic with a recently published book, *Coaching and Trauma* (2019).

Many therapists and counsellors will also have come across the work of Bessel van der Kolk and read his book *The Body Keeps the Score* (2015). This is part of a growing body of work that is showing the significance and prevalence of trauma in the lives of many who have witnessed or suffered abuse, much of it as children in the home – not just those who have suffered the most obvious traumas of war, conflict or physical injury. Ruppert and others go further, to define trauma in terms of the phenomena that are experienced by an individual, rather than what happens externally – in psychological terms, this casts splits in our personality as reactions to events, not the events themselves. Therefore *perceived* abandonment or emotional abuse, or even the fear of such things, might result in traumatic splitting. This brings us all within the scope of working with trauma and means that it is already in the coaching space, whether the coach and coachee are aware of it or not. This does not mean the psychosynthesis coach is going to work directly with healing the trauma in the way that a therapist might, but we do need to include an awareness of trauma within the scope of leadership coaching and an interest in the role of somatic work in healing such trauma. Some practitioners who have trained in somatic modalities might then explicitly combine healing work with coaching in appropriate ways.

For myself as a coach, I continue to grow in my awareness of the somatic perspective, simply by increasing my attention to body, posture and breath in the coaching space. Most of this takes place in terms of countertransference: through attending to my own body, posture and breath and using some of the somatic coaching questions listed above, I can sense or intuit what might be going on for the coachee.

Chapter 15

Coaching leaders in change, in crisis and towards synthesis

How does the psychosynthesis coach support leaders through change? When does change become crisis? How do we support leaders through crisis? How do we support leaders to create inner and outer synthesis through working with subpersonalities and the balance of opposites? How can we or our clients engage with synthesis as a transformational path in our lives?

Unpacking the topic of change

Change has been an enduring preoccupation of organisational development practitioners, certainly since I got involved in OD in the early 1990s. You might say that achieving successful *intentional* transformative change, whether at individual or collective levels, is the holy grail of our profession – desirable, mysterious, elusive, within our grasp and then lost again, with occasional standout successes. Pundits, gurus, consultants and coaches assure their audiences that, if you follow their advice, method or formula, you too can make the changes you want in your life, work or organisation. Personal experience and observational evidence mostly tells us it's not quite so simple. I will seek to create clarity around this big topic of change and then share an updated model of mindset change.

First, in a Wilberian kind of way, let's create some basic distinctions. Change is a fat word that refers to a vast sea of different things and we tend to use it indiscriminately. A primary distinction is between *intentional* and *unintentional* change; between change or transformation that we want to bring about and change that happens to us, unexpectedly, often undesirably, sometimes called disruptive change. Then, as already mentioned, there are *individual* and *collective* levels of change. So, intentional individual change might be about developing some personal capacity or skill (e.g. I want to be better at working with conflict) and intentional organisational change is often about shifting culture or mindsets (e.g. from a competitive to collaborative mindset). Disruptive individual change is often caused by an unwelcomed event (e.g. losing one's job, the breakdown of a relationship, a bereavement or illness), or by an unfolding inner crisis of meaning or duality (e.g. I don't see the point anymore). Disruptive change at the organisational level is often about a forced reaction to adverse performance or changing market conditions, or perhaps a change of ownership or a new strategy. Then there might be different degrees, magnitudes and timescales for change and transformation. Looking back at my life I can see a whole series of changes or developments that I didn't see at the time (e.g. how I have become less analytical and controlling and more intuitive and emergent).

Theories and models of change can help us with all of these different types of change in different ways, and most coaches will have their own repertoire to draw upon. A quick scan of my bookshelf reveals at least twenty books with 'change' in the title and there are many others with transformation or transition as their focus. To make some basic distinctions, there are change models that help us deal with unintentional change (e.g. Kubler-Ross's or Satir's model of change) and change models that are about making change happen (e.g. Kotter's eight steps, or countless NLP tools). I don't want to dwell too long on models that are not specific to psychosynthesis coaching, although I do want to touch on a couple before taking you into the psycho-synthesis approach to mindset change.

As a starting point, the leadership coach, or any type of coach for that matter, needs to understand the human process of change in response to unintentional change. On our coaching courses we introduce the Kubler-Ross change curve (adapted from her research on bereavement in *On Death and Dying*, 1969), as a widely acknowledged and accepted model for this, but we start by asking our students to reflect upon experiences of change in their lives and their reactions and responses to them. We always find that sharing these reflections together creates something like the Kubler-Ross model as a way of mapping what happens around change, particularly in organisational settings. The important part of this exercise lies in recognising the primacy of feelings and emotions in the process, and therefore the need for emotional awareness and maturity on the parts of both the coach and the coachee when working with the human process of change. Figure 15.1 features a version of the change curve I have worked with, including an illustration of how the locus of progress along the curve is usually different for leadership teams and the people they are leading.

One of the most popular recent approaches to facilitating intentional change is found in Robert Kegan and Lisa Lahey's *Immunity to Change*, first published in 2009. The essence of their model is that *competing commitments*, held in place by unquestioned assumptions or mindsets that lurk in our unconscious, may derail or block our conscious attempts to change our behaviour or transform ourselves. They develop their model using examples of individual and organisational change, weaving together the challenge of supporting transformation through the stages of their previously espoused developmental model of evolving cognitive complexity.

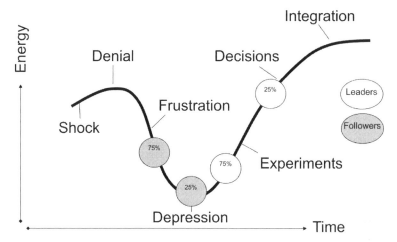

Figure 15.1 The Kubler-Ross (1969) change curve applied to an organisational change example.

The book is full of insights and I like the neatness of describing developmental progress in terms of *'making our subjective developmental stage an object of awareness, which allows us to work with it'*. However, I also found it a difficult book to read and concluded that there are both other developmental models and other change tools I prefer to work with. For anyone else having difficulty working their way through this book, I recommend a blog piece by William Harryman (2009), which summarises Kegan and Lahey's works to date and offers a simple step-by-step version of their change model for coaches. I resonate with Harryman's view that *'the idea of hidden assumptions and competing commitments really is nothing new for some of us – those who have been doing parts (subpersonalities) work for more than just a little while'*.

Kegan and Lahey (2009) make an important link between change, development and organisational culture: *'To foster real change and development, both the leader and the organisational culture **must take a developmental stance**, they must send the message that they expect adults can grow' (p308)*. They also refer to the age-old philosophical battle concerning personal change (p319):

Are we better off trying to reflect our way toward transformation, expecting eventual changes in behaviour as the outcome of our hardworking contemplation? Or would we be better off taking up new behaviours as best we can and trusting that our minds will catch up with the realities of our new experience?

Thus, they contrast the insight or depth approach to psychology with the behavioural modification approach, and point the way to transcending this dichotomy through *praxis* – '*practice specifically designed to explore the possibility of altering our personal and organisational theories' (p320),* (or big assumptions). This makes sense and follows the tradition of reflective practice as espoused by Chris Argyris and Donald Schon amongst others. However, I am left pondering the *cognitive-behavioural* bias that runs through Kegan and Lahey's work and the need to embrace systemic and somatic perspectives when approaching the challenge of change. This leads us to our preferred approach to enabling change for psychosynthesis coaches – *mindset change.*

Mindsets

I work with a model of **mindset change** adapted from one I first learnt about on the MA course in psychosynthesis psychology, and later used as a coach working with Roger Evans in Creative Leadership Consultants (the basics of which can be found in Roger Evans and Peter Russell's book *The Creative Manager*, 1989). There are similarities with the competing commitments model, in that our focus is to identity and become more conscious of limiting mindsets before seeking to reframe or transform them and change associated behaviour. Crucially, I now incorporate systemic and somatic perspectives as part of exploring and releasing the mindset, which I believe increases our chances of success.

The language of *mindsets* is becoming increasingly familiar within the organisational world, at both individual and collective levels. It is important to realise that we always have mindsets (beliefs, judgements, thought patterns, unconscious assumptions, etc.) and that it is our awareness of and relationship with them that we work on, with a view to giving ourselves more choice. The same mindset can be both empowering and limiting, healthy or dysfunctional, in different contexts or periods of our lives. As we grow and develop, the mindsets that helped us survive or succeed in the past may no longer serve us (e.g. '*don't rely upon others, I can do this on my own!*'). The same is true for collective mindsets: '*we are the best in the business!*' may serve the sales team at one point in time but can become limiting when the organisation needs to open up to collaborative partnerships. At the same time, some mindsets may point towards deeper psychological issues in our individual or collective psyches, and this is a theme which I will explore more fully in the future.

For now, here is the approach referred to above, which I have expanded to involve three parts, with ten steps.

Part one: identifying the mindset

1   What is the goal, purpose or agenda you want to work on? What blocks, barriers or issues are you experiencing in relationship to this (goal, purpose, agenda)? What are your observations, thoughts and feelings in

relation to these? Is this an issue that warrants deeper work to bring about change or transformation?

2   Explore limiting mindsets that you associate with this issue, block or barrier. These might be thought patterns or voices in your mind. Which of these feels the most significant? Which do you want to work with? Write down the mindset, being as specific as possible and using language which is familiar.

3   How does this mindset affect your behaviour and feelings? What behaviours do you associate with this mindset? What feelings do you associate with it?

Part two: unpacking the mindset

4   How strong is this mindset? In other words, how much does it control you, how automatic is it? How much choice do you have around it? (e.g. on a scale of 1-10, where 10 = completely automatic with no choice).

5   How long have you had this mindset? When and how did it first get started? Is there a time before that you can remember?

6   How does the mindset serve you? What do you get from it? What quality or value does it represent for you?

7   How does the mindset limit you? What does the mindset stop you from seeing or doing about yourself or about others?

Part three: reframing the mindset

8   How or where might this mindset be held in form, in your body? Can you put your hand there? Is there a shape or pattern to this mindset? Breathe into that place, and release.

9   In what ways is this mindset held in place, supported or perpetuated by the wider system of which you are part (e.g. family, organisation, society)? Which part of you is identified with this mindset? Which part(s) of you are not identified with the mindset and have choice in relationship to it?

10   As you step back from the mindset, what new space opens up within you? What new prospects does this open up for you? What freedom or choice do you have in terms of your behaviour? In what other ways might you meet the needs or commitment this mindset represented for you? Which empowering mindsets or affirmations could you draw upon in place of this mindset?

The relationship between *mindsets*, our *feelings* or emotional charge and our *behaviours* that are associated with them is depicted in Figure 15.2 above, which also shows how these are held in place through *form*. With individual mindsets this means the body or soma and related somatic patterns, and with collective or organisational mindsets this can be many different things, for

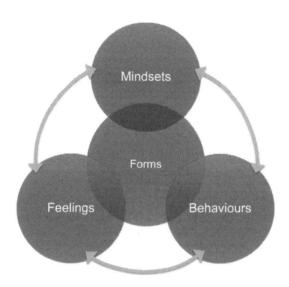

Figure 15.2 Mindsets in relationship with feelings, behaviours and forms.

example the formal and informal shapes and patterns of the organisational system and its culture.

I always offer coaches a word of warning about this kind of work: mindsets are slippery, and finding the mindset that needs working on in relation to a purpose, goal or issue is a serious challenge in itself. The coach's task is to help the client self-reflect and increase their self-awareness in ways that they would not otherwise manage to do. Finding an important mindset to work with may take time – more than one session. It may help to suggest that the client keeps a journal and records thought processes between sessions, as close as possible in real time to significant events or patterns of behaviour they want to change. You are trying to help the client catch their inner negative or critical voices and externalise them by putting them into words. It is surprising how often these turn out to be words used by a critical parent or authority figure or perhaps a resonant expression from the client's childhood. I take notes during coaching sessions and will capture phrases spoken by the coachee that might be these familiar thought patterns or mindsets and then ask the client about them at an appropriate time, for example when working in the gap to address a block or barrier. If the client recognises the phrase as an important mindset, this can then lead into more in-depth work.

Referring back to our model of interventions in Chapter 8, exploring mindsets is one way to work at depth with the coachee; the subpersonalities model of the psyche is another. We briefly discussed in Chapter 8 how the psychosynthesis coach might follow one of these different approaches depending upon the language or other cues given by the coachee. We now briefly turn our attention to the subpersonalities approach.

Subpersonalities

One of the most harmful illusions that can beguile us is probably the belief that we are an indivisible, immutable, totally consistent being. And finding out that the contrary is true is among the first tasks – and possible surprises – that confronts us in the adventure of our psychosynthesis.

Piero Ferrucci (1982, p47)

"There are times," said Somerset Maugham, "when I look over the various parts of my character with perplexity. I recognise that I am made up of several persons and that the person that at the moment has the upper hand will inevitably give place to another."

(Quoted in TA Harris, 1969, p1; Requoted in J Evans, 2009)

The approach we use for working with subpersonalities on our courses is based upon that taught by the Institute of Psychosynthesis (J Evans, 2009). We introduce the five-stage model of subpersonality harmonisation (recognition-acceptance-coordination-integration-synthesis) to our coaching students on our PGCPLC courses. In addition, in leadership coaching, we can combine subpersonalities work in a variety of different ways by working at individual, group and organisation levels with our clients. For example I often use Belbin Team Roles profiling (Belbin, 2004) with individuals and teams and the various team roles (Plant, Resource Investigator, Coordinator, Shaper, Monitor Evaluator, Teamworker, Implementer, Specialist) can be used as a shared language of archetypal organisational subpersonalities within team coaching. As another example, we can help our leadership clients look at how they might adapt the five stages of subpersonality harmonisation to both leadership teams and working with the different parts of the organisation as a whole.

The psychosynthesis coach might not always explicitly introduce the model of subpersonalities, but can nevertheless draw upon the principles outlined below to work with them. I often do this, referring to the parts of ourselves rather than subpersonalities. Coachees may naturally refer to parts of themselves in relationship to their thinking, feelings and behaviours, so we might ask them to tell us more about that part of themselves. That is often the start of this work.

I would also add that we view subpersonalities as an inner systemic model of the psyche, in which all the elements are in a complex and forever-changing inter-relationship and in further complex relationships with systems beyond the individual psyche. Therefore, when engaged with systemic constellations work as described in Chapter 12, we might naturally combine this with subpersonalities or parts work when working with the inner world of the client.

To provide the reader new to subpersonalities with a basic introduction, I include the following edited text by Paul Elliott, which draws from material provided on the aforementioned Institute of Psychosynthesis programmes (J Evans, 2009).

During the last one hundred years, this inner complexity has been a major theme of psychology. From the time of William James (who according to Assagioli called subpersonalities 'the various selves'), psychologists have recognised the importance of the divisions within our psyche and the corresponding psychological formation that results from them.

Once we turn our attention to them we find many subpersonalities within each of us. Some are common to many of us (father, mother, son, daughter, teacher, manager, critic, coach, rebel, pleaser etc.) but others are more unique – the more so by our identifying and recognising them and naming them (naming is very important because it identifies the subpersonality in relation to our own particular psyche).

Subpersonalities exist within a multiplex of other subpersonalities perhaps working in harmony with others, but often in opposing pairs or in complex patterns of inter-relationship.

Subpersonalities form as a synthesis of habit patterns, traits, complexes and other psychological elements. But in order to have a synthesis, there has to be a centre around which the synthesis occurs. In a subpersonality, this centre is an inner drive or urge that strives to be realised. It is this centre that attracted and synthesised various personality elements to create what can be considered as its own body or its own means of expression.

As we gradually recognise and harmonise them, they in turn become organised and synthesised around a higher order centre which is the 'I' – the personal centre of identity.

This higher order synthesis becomes the integrated personality – the harmonious and effective means of expression of the self-actualised human being. As we move towards this goal, we become increasingly able to choose at any moment which subpersonality we wish to express. *Until then we can be controlled by whichever subpersonality that we unconsciously identify with in the moment and thus limited by its particular attributes.*

Often subpersonalities form at a young age as a survival mechanism to gain acceptance and love in our family of origin. So, for example a pleaser subpersonality could develop as a child experiences that he/

she does not receive unconditional from their parents but can get love by adapting their behaviour. What starts as an essential survival mechanism becomes an unconscious default mode which may severely limit the adult. Taking the example further, as the child moves to adolescence and starts to individuate then a rebel subpersonality might develop and then there will be two opposing subpersonalities.

In coaching, working with a coachee's subpersonalities can be an extremely useful way of helping them develop their self-awareness and therefore find where their will is caught. In doing so the client and the coach can potentially identify more clearly where the coachee's will is available to make changes to their personal and professional lives.

The key point is that subpersonalities of which we are not aware can control us and limit our capacity to choose. What we are unconscious of controls us. This is also the core learning about identification and disidentification. In order to disidentify we must first identify – bring to consciousness, then we have the power to choose.

Reproduced by kind permission of The Institute of Psychosynthesis, London, 2020

The process or method for working with subpersonalities involves five stages – recognition, acceptance, coordination, integration and synthesis – and these can be summarised as below. In practice, the leadership coach might informally work through all of these stages within a single session or may find they work through them over several sessions.

Process of harmonisation of subpersonalities – the 5-stage model

1. **Recognition**: subpersonalities develop unconsciously. Initially during this stage we develop awareness as to how they operate and see how they shape our view of ourselves and the world. The more the individual becomes conscious of the parts, the more the sense of 'I-ness' – the one who chooses – develops. Within the complexity of 'I am this, that and the other' comes 'I am all this – I am myself'.

2. **Acceptance:** this stage is devoted to seeing 'what is' without value judgement. This is often difficult, as the subpersonality may be an aspect of the person that they don't like and have repressed. The more it is repressed, the more it asserts itself. Acceptance can be a journey of understanding the subpersonality's likely origins, as well as the way that it has served in the past and the qualities that it

includes that may serve the present and future. When working with subpersonalities at this acceptance stage (and also at the next coordination stage), it is useful to in turn describe the subpersonality's behaviour, identify its wants and its needs and finally recognise its qualities.

3. **Coordination:** whenever we go deep enough towards the core of a subpersonality, we find that the core – which is some basic urge or need – is good. For practical purposes this can be considered an absolute. No matter how many layers of distortion surround it, the basic need, the basic motivation is a good one – and if it becomes twisted that is because of not being able to express itself directly. The real core – not what the subpersonality wants but what it needs – is good. A basic purpose of the coordination stage is to discover this central urge or need, to make it conscious and to find acceptable ways it can be satisfied and fulfilled.

4. **Integration:** while coordination deals with the development and improvement within each subpersonality, integration is concerned with the relationship with other subpersonalities and with each one's place and activity within the personality as a whole. The process of integration leads from a general state of isolation, conflict, competition and repression of the weaker elements by the strong ones, to a state of harmonious cooperation in which the effectiveness of the personality is greatly enhanced. It's useful then when working as a coach to look at a coachee's subpersonalities' relationship with each other. This could be a helpful route to identifying available will.

5. **Synthesis**: this final stage represents a potential move from intrapersonal development as represented by integration to interpersonal and transpersonal development. Synthesis is an outcome of a growing interplay of the personality with the superconscious and the transpersonal Self. As a result of this interplay, the life of the individual and their interaction with other human beings becomes increasingly characterised by a sense of responsibility, caring, harmonious cooperation, altruistic love and transpersonal objectives. It leads to the harmonious integration of the human being with others, with mankind and with the world.

Reproduced by kind permission of the Institute of Psychosynthesis, London, 2020

The topic of subpersonalities is introduced on most basic introductory psychosynthesis programmes, although it features more strongly in the training of some schools than others. We would warn against the over-use of this approach in coaching simply because it seems an easy way to create awareness and generate energy with clients. My advice is to be critical, selective and reflective about explicitly introducing any technique or intervention in coaching rather than following the natural engagement with what is already in the coaching space, alongside maintaining our central focus on working with Self and Will as described in the method of trifocal vision.

I have observed some students becoming too caught up in the excitement of this work and, having identified their subpersonalities, becoming more identified with them rather than less. We need to stay connected with the larger context for this work of identification and disidentification, leading to a strengthening of the coachee's experience of the 'I' and capacity for self-awareness.

Working with crisis in coaching

When does change become crisis? How do we support leaders through crisis?

This is a tricky, complex but important topic, which we can only just start to address within the scope of this book. As psychosynthesis coaches we need to be aware of and able to acknowledge crisis in the lives of our clients. At the same time, the way in which we might work with crisis will depend much upon our training and professional experience, as well as our own personal development and experience.

The standard response of many executive coaches to encountering a significant existential crisis is to refer the client to a therapist or other specialist. This might not be an option, not least because many leaders are not willing to enter therapy, although they are happy to work with a coach. Therefore the coaching relationship may be the only form of help or support available to the leader during their time of crisis. For the most part, having someone that they trust, with whom they can talk in confidence and who will listen without judgement, can make an enormous difference. Then there is at least a chance that the coachee will take the risk to talk about what is really going on for them.

It helps to distinguish between the different types and levels of crisis we might come across. The term *crisis* is frequently used to describe the state of affairs in our outer lives, in the organisations we work within and in society at large and, in this sense, crisis is an increasing prevalent condition. Some organisations and their leaders appear to be in a permanent state of crisis, although this is often a pathological condition. There are natural crises of transition as an organisation grows and develops, for example between the paradigms or worldviews described in Chapter 13.

As psychosynthesis practitioners we are more concerned with inner crisis in our lives, which may or may not be related to or co-exist with an outer crisis. Most importantly, the psychosynthesis perspective on inner existential crisis is that it is a natural occurrence in the process of personal and spiritual growth and something to recognise, understand and work with, rather than deny, be ashamed of or get rid of. There are many different types of crisis and we must be wary of generalising, but we are primarily concerned with recognising crisis as a symptom of our higher Self seeking a way to be expressed – of a release or frustration of higher energies from our superconscious. The source of this crisis is therefore our transpersonal Self or superconscious, rather than our lower unconscious, and this is what distinguishes these experiences from psychological pathologies that originate from our wounding or trauma in the past. An added difficulty surrounding this is that sometimes crisis can be experienced as debilitating and involving enormous suffering, and at other times as liberating and accompanied by an outpouring of higher energies. Much also depends upon the ego strength of the person experiencing crisis, as well as the co-existence of latent or active lower-unconscious pathologies that might complicate the crisis. The picture can quickly become complicated and the temptation to simply refer the problem elsewhere is understandable.

Self-realisation and self-actualisation: crises of duality and meaning

However, I return to the most common situation wherein the leadership coach encounters explicit or implicit evidence of crisis and where the options to refer elsewhere are unrealistic. To simplify the picture, we return to the model of self-actualisation and self-realisation we introduced in Chapter 3 and revisited in Chapter 11 on leadership development (and see Figure 15.3).

We use this model to highlight the two most common types of existential crisis:

- The crisis of **meaning**, experienced by *actualisers* – when they reach a point of personal doubt, meaninglessness or spiritual aridity in their previously driven, unquestioned or confident lives.
- The crisis of **duality**, experienced by *transcenders* – when they return from spiritual exploration or experiences of self-realisation to find the real world too painful or difficult to deal with and are significantly challenged to make their lives work.

As John Whitmore describes in *Coaching for Performance* (4th edition, 2009), the former is the crisis most commonly encountered in executive coaching, when under the stresses and pressures of leadership we lean too far to the self-actualisation side, *'we are liable eventually to run into a wake-up call wall. This is known as the crisis of meaning'*. Whitmore goes on to describe what this might look like and advocates that coaches who want to support leaders through such crises should seek some form of training in psychosynthesis.

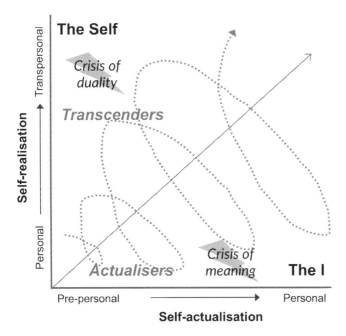

Figure 15.3 Two dimensions of self-development – and the crises of meaning and duality.

As Whitmore comments, not all psycho-spiritual development involves disruptive or disturbing crises of meaning or duality – everyone is following their unique journey, and some will choose to journey further than others. However, I would suggest that everyone will benefit in some way from a coach who is aware of the psycho-spiritual dimension of development and attuned to the resonances of the Self seeking expression. Many people have experienced some form of spiritual awakening through peak experiences but never spoken about them or made sense of their meaning, and the psychosynthesis coach can offer the opportunity for this level of inner reflection.

Assagioli's four-stage model of spiritual awakening

It helps to have some kind of road map for what a crisis of meaning/spiritual awakening looks like, and Assagioli provides this in Chapter 2 of *Psychosynthesis* (1965), on 'Self-realisation and psychological disturbances'. His work is ground-breaking, and he was the first depth psychologist to deeply understand the context and process of self-awakening and realisation. Many followed (e.g. Grof), building upon this core platform of work.

Table 15.1 Symptoms of psychological disturbance (examples, not exhaustive)

Crisis preceding awakening	Crisis of awakening
• Aridity	• Bliss
• Boredom	• Dissociation
• Change	• Extreme emotion
• Crisis of meaning	• Fear of death
• Depression	• Intense shyness
• Mania	• Overwhelm
• Meaning of suffering	• Psychosis
• Meaninglessness	• Repression of sublime
• Repression of sublime	• Terror
• Self-doubt	• Transcendence
Reactions to awakening	**Integration**
• Crisis of duality	• Dealing with past obstacles
• Dark night of soul	• Down to earth
• Depression	• Frustration
• Fanaticism	• Holding/embracing difference
• Idealisation	• Humility
• Inflation	• Ordinariness
• Overwhelm	• Pain of reality
• Schizoid	• Suffering aspiration/reality
• Splitting	• Suffering meaning
• Unreality	• Working through

For those interested in exploring this topic further I would direct you to read this chapter from Assagioli. Otherwise, here is a simple summary of Assagioli's four-stage model of spiritual awakening and an illustration of the symptoms that might help the coach recognise clients experiencing these stages:

1 Crisis preceding awakening (life lacks meaning)
2 Crisis of awakening (things may never be the same again, you can't hold things in the same way)
3 Reactions to awakening (e.g. inflation and mystic flight or denial and suppression)
4 Integration (grounding, bringing energies down into the personal from the transpersonal)

Life stages and developmental stages

Crisis can also be differentiated in terms of life stages. The most commonly identified are in adolescence (leading to an inflated sense of self) and in mid-life (leading to a deflated sense of self). At the Institute of Psychosynthesis Joan Evans has developed a model that highlights the crises experienced at each turn of the spiral in the process of individuation:

Characteristics of each turn of the spiral

Birth: I am – Physical separation with the cutting of the umbilical cord

Adolescence: I am that – Emotional separation bringing about the existential experience of worthlessness. Using emotional energy – anger – to separate; using the will to serve the building of autonomy, and the mind to justify separation. Creating forms in the world for the expression of individuality.

Mid-life: I am that I am – Separation from the personality – concrete mind. Using the will to separate from the mind. Pulling back consciousness from outer forms (i.e. belief systems, rationalisations for identifications). Dealing with 'temptations' of the world and letting go of attachments.

(J Evans, 2009)

Picking up on a theme we touched upon in Chapter 11, I have started to do some work to map the different crises that might be associated with making transitions between paradigms or developmental stages.

We must recognise that some people experience relatively little transition between developmental stages in their lives (horizontal developers) and some experience relatively frequent and disruptive changes (vertical developers). There are therefore two different ways to read a developmental stages profile (e.g. the LDF or leadership styles profiles mentioned in Chapter 13): (i) as a relatively stable and constant description of your leadership paradigm, worldview or value systems make-up; or (ii) as a guide to the tensions and transitions between value systems that are taking place within you. If you experience relative stability, consistency and satisfaction in your life, it may be the former; if you are experiencing some form of inner crisis (e.g. stress, change, uncertainty, loss of confidence, direction or meaning, etc.), it may well be the latter. The table below describes some of the possible elements and aspects of the different stages of transition between value systems, which you may recognise from different periods within your life.

This model is purely a hypothesis based upon my own personal and professional experience and needs testing and validation. Collaborators are welcome.

Conclusion

As I said at this start of this section, this is a complex topic which we can only just touch upon within the scope of this book. The wider territory of spiritual emergence and emergency, along with understanding how to distinguish between existential and neurotic shame and guilt, are covered well elsewhere

Table 15.2 Crises at transition points between stages of development

Leadership style/paradigm + Graves mode	Crisis	Signs	Examples
Benevolent-Magic Animistic →	Crisis of Will 1: Expression	Need to break away from the parental hold, find your voice, be yourself.	Terrible twos Adolescent acting out Hero's journey – setting out
Autocratic-Impulsive Egocentric →	Crisis of Self 1: Truth	There has to be more to life than this. Neurotic guilt and shame. Search for some higher meaning or truth.	Seeing the light Reforming your ways Commitment to a discipline or path
Hierarchical-Conformist Absolutist →	Crisis of Will 2: Actualisation	Disenchantment with authority. Old ways no longer work. Knowing you can do it better, wanting to realise your potential.	Setting up on your own or seeking advancement Leaving your mentor behind Breaking the rules to improve
Enterprising-Achievement Multiplistic →	Crisis of Self 2: Meaning	There has to be more to life than this. Existential guilt and shame. Loss of confidence or motivation. Loss of meaning or direction.	Classic mid-life crisis acting out Emotional or cathartic release Starting an inner journey or path of discovery

Social-Pluralistic *Relativistic* →	Crisis of Will 3: Difference	Frustrated by pluralistic mindset. Existential crisis. Experiencing paradox and synchronicity. Finding new ways that work.	Letting go of control and going with the present-centred flow. Complex or systemic thinking. Release of heightened creativity
Integrative-Evolutionary *Systemic* →	Crisis of Self 3: Purpose	Loss of old, changing identity. Experiencing universal love and acceptance. Connection with global or higher energies.	Self-reflective practices. Increasing focus on others. Building global community and connections
Holistic-Evolutionary *Holistic*			

(e.g. Simpson et al., 2013). However, the coach who is serious about working at this level with a client requires significant personal and professional development and in-depth training of some kind; as an example, starting with one of the psychosynthesis introductory short courses on offer, such as the 'Fundamentals of psychosynthesis' at the Institute for Psychosynthesis or the 'Essentials' at the Psychosynthesis Trust in London.

Coaching towards synthesis of opposites

At the heart of much of the change or crisis that we experience in our lives is the continuous process of emergent growth, driven by the evolutionary principle of tension between dichotomous opposites, seeking synthesis. Working more essentially and at greater depth with change and crisis leads us to engage with this evolutionary principle of synthesis at multiple levels. This perhaps represents the zenith of working as a psychosynthesis coach and as such, in our search for mastery, we are continuously learning and practising the principles that I will attempt to outline briefly in this section.

Roberto Assagioli wrote a couple of papers (which resided in the archives at Casa Assagioli in Florence and were recently translated into English by my friend and colleague Gordon Symons) that I have found enormously helpful with understanding how to work with synthesis as a coach. Of course, Assagioli has written about synthesis elsewhere, including in *The Act of Will* (1974), and most books on psychosynthesis include something about the principles or process of synthesis. Of these, I recommend Petra Guggisberg Nocelli's Chapter VI in Part Four of *The Way of Psychosynthesis* (2017) as a next step in understanding this theme.

The first of the two papers I refer to is 'Unity in Diversity' (2018, np), in which he describes this key principle:

> In order to establish proper relations between human beings and human groups, it is necessary to understand, accept and practise a great principle or truth, which is at the basis of life itself in all its manifestations: that of UNITY IN DIVERSITY
> …the true nature of this unity must be well understood and applied. Unity should not be understood as uniformity and absence of any differentiation, but in a functional, dynamic and organic sense.
> The relations between the substantial unity and the boundless multiplicity are regulated – as far as we are given to know – by two great principles: Polarity and Diversity of functions.

He then goes on to explain what he means by *diversity of functions* (e.g. why we need different personality types in a team) before directing us to the second paper to understand how we can work with *polarity*.

This paper, on the 'Balance and the Synthesis of Opposites' (which has been used for some time by our IIPE colleagues in Italy), also starts out with some basic principles:

> It is good to clarify from the beginning that every polarity is a relationship between two elements and that, as such, it is never absolute, but relative to that given pair of terms. Therefore, the same element can be positive with respect to a given 'pole', and negative with respect to another.

So polarity is not about absolutes of good and bad, but something more dynamic. Assagioli shows that, once we start to look, we can see polarities operating everywhere, for example in the human personality – important ones he mentions include psyche–body, unconscious–conscious, receptive–active, introversion–extraversion, intuitive–sensory, inspiration–aspiration, heart–mind. I recently identified five key polarities to observe and hold in our awareness as coaches working with our clients: unconscious–conscious; inner–outer; individual–collective; wholes–parts; self-realisation–self-actualisation. What I look for here is some evidence of movement or flow between the polarities as a sign of healthy personal development and emergent Self.

Thus we start to realise that the polarity of opposites is at the heart of most tension and disturbance in our lives and human affairs in general, as well the path and progress of evolution, or conversely the path of regression and breakdown/destruction (as we are experiencing in the current global political climate).

For the leadership coach or facilitator, I highlight five principles to engage with before working directly with a client towards the resolution of polar tension towards synthesis.

1   The first is to be curious, inquiring and reflective about which polarity it is that you should be working with. Have you and the coachee identified the right polarity to work with? As an example, typically coaches tend to work with clients on the so-called work–life balance, but often on closer inspection this might become something like family–career, or even self-actualisation versus self-realisation. David Whyte has written a fascinating book called *The Three Marriages* (2009) in which he examines the balance and tensions between the polarities in our lives of *self*, *work* and *relationship*, and explores how we might create synthesis between each of these, bringing them into higher alignment (rather than a horizontal balance or compromise).
2   The second is to observe how the polarity shows up in terms of the awareness, goals, stories, concerns and issues that the coachee brings to coaching. As we observed in Chapter 3, some coachees might talk only about their outer lives, others might talk mainly about their inner lives.

As mentioned above, we are looking for signs of some engagement or movement and flow of energies between the polarities, rather than stuckness at one end and blindness at the other.

3   The third is to be curious, inquiring and reflective about how the polar tension is externalising or playing out in terms of thoughts, feelings and behaviours for the coachee. This might include identifying related mindsets or subpersonalities that are part of this polarity.

4   The fourth is to observe what is conscious and what is unconscious (for the coachee) – is this a polarity tension that they are aware of, that is a continuing struggle in their lives, or it is something underlying which they have not brought fully to consciousness?

5   The fifth is to notice where the attention is focused in the polarity, and which of the polar opposites might need more attention, perhaps just in terms of being named or articulated. Often this is all that is needed to shift the energy and resolve the tension.

We have already touched upon some of the different levels at which we might work with polarities. The psychosynthesis leadership coach might work with synthesis at any or all of these levels:

- In our inner selves – for example feeling and thinking, imagination and desire, intuition and sensation, realisation and actualisation.
- In our personal lives – for example safety and exploration, self and others, career and family, past and future.
- In organisations – for example stability and change, individual and team, development and performance, belonging and growth.
- In society – for example conservation and progress, individual and collective identity, freedom and security, local and global.

Before we embark upon a method of working with polarity with our clients it is important that we have worked in this way on ourselves, and I would suggest that the psychosynthesis coach should explore the tensions in their lives at each of the above levels. To give a brief personal example, I have been working with the *mind–heart* polarity for many years (and have referred to this elsewhere in this book), which I experienced as a deep split in my personality (between my mind-identified survival self and my part-traumatised/part-healthy emotional self, buried subconsciously but able to respond when safe). I have recently experienced a synthesis between the two, resulting in an emergence of what I will call compassionate wisdom. There is now more flow and fusion between my intellect and my emotions; I feel they can be simultaneously present as I work professionally, rather than lurching from one to the other. I experience this not as a compromise between the mind and heart, but as the emergence of a new identity or energy altogether that works alchemically in new ways and is writing this book.

I will now introduce an approach to synthetic working involving six steps, as described to me by Alessandra Moretti (IIPE, 2019) at a recent retreat in France.

1 Recognising – seeing with new eyes for the first time
2 Accepting – without prejudice and judgement
3 Giving expression to the polarities
4 Understanding the needs of each polarity
5 Valuing the essential qualities and potentialities
6 Bringing about synthesis through balancing opposites to find new solutions and outcomes

There are similarities to the psychosynthesis way of working with subpersonalities here (which of course is also about working towards synthesis). To engage with the last of these steps in greater detail, we return to the source material of 'Balance and the Synthesis of Opposites' (Assagioli, 2018b).

Synthetic working to create synthesis between polarities – balancing opposites

The main outcomes and the main solutions of a 'polar tension' can be:

1. Fusion of the two poles, with the consequent neutralization of their energy charges.
2. Reabsorption of one of the poles into the other through the action of an 'intermediate centre', or of a principle superior to both.
3. The creation of a new being, of a new reality.
4. The regulation of opposite poles through the action of an 'intermediate centre'. This regulatory action can take place in two ways:
   a) By decreasing the amplitude of the oscillations, sometimes even to nullify them, thus producing a more or less complete neutralization.
   b) By directing the alternatives in a conscious and wise way, so that they have appropriate and constructive effects, in harmony with the cyclic alternations of the particular and general conditions, human and cosmic. (This is the method taught by Chinese philosophy and particularly by the I Ching, already mentioned).
5. Synthesis, through the work of a higher element or principle that transforms, sublimates and reabsorbs the two poles in a higher and wider reality.

(Assagioli, 2018b, np)

A student commented at a recent workshop that these options appear to ascend from the simplest possible outcomes to those involving most complexity. This method and material require far more explanation, unpacking and examples than I am able to provide here – another topic for my next book, on evolutionary leadership. However, I would like to end this section with an example of how this way of working with synthesis applies at a societal level, by returning to the first paper ('Unity in Diversity'). Here Assagioli (2018a, np) offers a very valuable insight that makes sense of many of the tensions and struggles in global politics and society in today:

> ...living humanity requires at least a mutual adjustment of the two tendencies. I said 'at least', because 'the balancing of the opposite poles' is not accomplished only through their mutual moderating action 'horizontally', on the same level, so to speak. In many cases it can be implemented even better by the intervention of a regulatory principle operating from a higher plane and with higher and more powerful energies than those in play and in conflict.
>
> In the present case, this Higher Principle consists of a synthetic and spiritual conception of history as the unfolding of human evolution towards a higher Goal, from the intuitive vision of a divine Plan. In this conception the intellectual, moral, aesthetic and social 'values' achieved in the past are not disowned but are freed from old forms which are no longer adequate, are re-experienced and re-expressed in different ways and adherent to the present, and integrated with the new 'values' conquered by the progressive consciousness of humanity.
>
> It can also be said that the proportions between conservative forces and innovative forces must not always be the same, but can and must vary according to historical periods.

The principles articulated here by Assagioli seem to me to be essential learning for societal leaders and politicians, regardless of where they might place their own preferred position along the polarity of *conservative–progressive*. Maybe I am being naïve, but seeking to engage our future leaders in this kind of education seems a good place to start with finding the way out of the current collective mess we find ourselves in.

Finally, it is interesting to reflect upon one of the polarities at the organisational level in a similar way – that of *stability* and *change*. The dominant paradigm in organisations over the last twenty to thirty years has been so heavily weighted towards the imperatives of the *change* polarity, to the neglect of the needs of the *stability* end, that I think it has caused much collateral damage. As part of the organisational change profession, I was very much implicated in this for many years. In hindsight I feel that we were mostly asking the wrong basic questions; for example instead of *'how do we bring about transformational change in this situation?'* it might have been better to ask *'what is the dynamic tension between change and stability in this situation and what new synthesis will transcend this?'*

A coaching story: *Supervision conversation*

Supervisor: Who do you see, when you open your heart to Michael?

Coach: Someone very driven by his deep sense of purpose, finding himself in a troubling, emotional place, wanting to make changes in his life but unable to take his foot off the relentless pressure to drive his organisation.

Supervisor: Where exactly is he struggling; where is he caught?

Coach: On one hand there's stress and grief in his family system, which I see as a catalyst for his personal process. On another hand he's having difficult conversations at work as he seeks to share responsibility and empower his people. But he keeps being let down and then doubts whether he can trust them, so he takes back the controls. This is all forcing him to reflect upon his drives and obsessions, the way he works and what he really wants in his life.

Supervisor: What is the big gap here?

Coach: Finding a way to transition to a way of working that doesn't sacrifice his own needs and those of his family. I suspect there is an unconscious fear that in doing this he might somehow lose the passion that led him to create this extraordinary project. He needs to have patience, accept that not everyone can operate to his amazing level and let people find their own way without jumping in. Then he can support and nurture the progress they are making and focus on what he's really good at, creating the vision, inspiring people to join and contribute to the project.

Supervisor: What might be the small gap, the next steps that he can take?

Coach: In his organisation he's putting in place leadership development and career paths for his people and running a series of team workshops. He can think about where he might let others take the lead with some of the sessions. He can then notice every time he wants to jump in and take charge, and ask himself whether he really needs to. We can work on the part of himself that needs to do that and where it comes from.

Supervisor: Where are you now in relationship to this coaching?

Coach: I am still feeling somewhat in awe of his brilliance and not sure what I contribute to him.

Supervisor: Where else might this be going on?

Coach: I can see that this is what his people might be feeling too.

Supervisor: Why do you think he found you as a coach?

Coach: I sense he wants a mirror to reflect back to him, as well as a guide to help him find a way through. A Virgil to his Dante I suppose.

Chapter 16

Coaching the Will

How does Assagioli's approach to developing the Will help leaders today? In what ways was his introspective scientific research decades ahead of today's experimental psychology and neuroscience? How might we work at greater depth to develop the Will with our clients?

The new determinism and the loss of free will

As we have previously said, psychosynthesis is a psychospiritual psychology of Self and Will. I would assert that psychosynthesis is the only fully developed psychology of Will because, with psychosynthesis, we focus on will rather than motivation and behaviour (which is what most conventional psychology is concerned with). This is because Will is both essential to our being (as the first expression of Self) and central to our psychological functioning. Max Landsberg, Graham Alexander and John Whitmore didn't choose Will as the W of GROW by accident (although other coaching manuals often reduce this W to *what* or *way*, thus losing the essence of the model). I would argue that Will is even more important to coaching and leadership today than it was in the 1980s when the aforementioned wise men first developed the GROW model.

Why is this the case? Expanding upon the discussion about free will and the existential crisis of leadership in Chapter 4, I would argue that an insidious new determinism is gaining hold in the collective psyche, with a corresponding sense of the loss of free will. I would point to the recent growth of populist politics as a symptom of this encroaching systemic loss, erosion and denial of free will as people experience an increasing sense of helplessness or loss of agency in a complex and confusing world. Within this context, one is attracted to charismatic and egotistical leaders who promise to take action and make things happen on our behalf, even if the action is a regressive and destructive smash (and grab what they can for themselves) of the old order without putting anything constructive in its place.

How did this new determinism take hold and what can we do about it? It helps to start by recognising it. I offer these perspectives to help with that:

- **Wilber's 'Flatland'** – colonisation of inner realm by scientific materialism
  Ken Wilber's concept of Flatland, as described in many of his works (e.g. 2000), provides a clear philosophical and historical explanation of what has been happening in terms of the growing domination of the scientific paradigm over recent decades. With reference to his four quadrants model (which we introduced in Chapter 13), he defines *"Flatland – or scientific materialism – as the belief that only matter (or matter/energy) is real, and that only* narrow science *has any claim to truth. (Narrow science, recall, is the science of any Right-Hand domain, whether that be atomistic science of the Upper Right, or systems science of the Lower Right.) Flatland, in other words, is the belief that only the Right-Hand quadrants are real."* (Wilber, 2000, np) The consequence is a world in which everything is reduced to surfaces and there is no acknowledgement of depth.
- **Neuroscience and neuropsychology** – the all-powerful unconscious
  In Chapter 4 we looked at how neuropsychology has contributed to the new determinism, and we will expand our understanding of what neuropsychology has to tell us in Chapter 18. The thrust of what much neuroscience is telling us is that we are not as in control as we think, and that most of what we do is determined by the unconscious functioning of the brain.
- **Genetics and evolutionary psychology** – we are our biology
  These are fields of research related to neuroscience that go a step further in telling us that much of the unconscious functioning of the brain is determined by our sex, biology and genetic programming from hundreds of thousands of years of evolutionary history. As an example, the 'What science is telling us' page in *The Week* flows with new discoveries and stories about how we are pre-programmed by our genetic and evolutionary history.
- **Social media and big data** – all-encompassing behavioural predictability
  Coming into the present day, we have a particular set of problems resulting from technological developments that in the last twenty years have changed the way the world works so rapidly that only corporate behemoths, smart entrepreneurs, manipulative opportunists and unscrupulous criminals seem to have worked out how to operate in the new reality to their advantage. The mass of the population who have become beholden to mobile technology, social media and interactive everything act as unconscious puppets to the ensuing constant communications (or nudges) driven by the undeclared motives of others. Those entrusted with protecting society or guarding civilisation have become so outflanked and outmanoeuvred that they don't know which way to turn and so do

nothing, or not enough. Of course, looked at from the corporate perspective, big data that increasingly invades and absorbs every aspect of our lives gives the new masters of the universe an unerring control over how people behave. 1984 has arrived, and no one noticed.

- **Consumerism and stimulus addiction** – sensory overwhelm society
Taking the picture above to the individual psychological level, our valency for or vulnerability to addiction has found a whole new set of outlets within this new epoch. These include not just all of social media, in whatever flavour you find acceptable or like best; for leaders and anyone working in organisations the domination of emails and computers work likewise; so do our mobile phones and all their apps; gaming, gambling and other potentially dark habits that increasingly can be accessed on any platform you might like; and alternative worlds and virtual reality that appears to know no potential bounds. The need for constant sensory or external stimulation is becoming an individual and collective psychological problem of significant proportions. Social media experts talk about click-ability and clickbait as the mechanisms by which this 'attention economy' operates. For example I know I am addicted to the chemical hits I get from checking my emails far too often, or from the sports scores or the news headlines on my phone, unconsciously hoping for a little boost to my mood but equally vulnerable to deflationary pinpricks. Combine all this with the (particularly British) addictions to consumerism, celebrity and borrowing cash that were already well fed by the old media of TV and newspapers, and we have a heady concoction that is making addiction therapists working with traditional substance and relationship addictions even busier than they already were. Brave New World has arrived, and no one noticed.
- **VUCA world** – an overwhelming environment where we have no control
We have already well illustrated in Chapter 4 how VUCA manifests. VUCA stands for *volatility, uncertainty, complexity* and *ambiguity*. Quoting Keith Silvester and Heather Wignall on the origins of this very useful term (Symposium paper 2018): *"It draws originally on the leadership theories of W Bennis and B Nanus, and was developed by Ron Heifetz and Marty Linsky under the more generally known term 'Adaptive Leadership'. As a term beloved by the American military, VUCA is now widely used to encapsulate the conditions under which organisational systems have to operate and make decisions in a postmodern world."* Silvester and Wignall went on to show in a workshop how each of the VUCA elements can be approached from a psycho-spiritual perspective, to start to give us a way of navigating through this overwhelming environment.
- **Systems within systems** – how much choice do we have?
Recent developments in organisational theory, for example complexity theory, developmental psychology and systemic coaching (supported

scientifically by neuropsychology, as mentioned above), have made enormous gains in helping us understand why things are the way they are and how they change and evolve over time, but they also have the collective impact of marginalising individual free will. If the system, or the culture, or the paradigm, or the unconscious is so powerful and all pervasive, what chance do we have of exercising free choice and individual agency?

From her recent EFPP workshop, which I attended, Kristina Brode (workshop handout, 2019) sums this all up rather well;

> Free will a fairy tale? Neurosciences could make us believe this. Are we really run by archaic programs and unconscious prejudices? That life would be nothing more than millions of reflexive reactions. Looking around the world it seems we are reigned by – our fear of the foreign, strange or unknown and our longing for be-longing.

She goes on to requote Joan Evans: *"Unwittingly, therefore, we live our lives through the magnetic pull of the historical past which seems to have a will of its own despite our very best intentions"*.

What can we do about it?

Of course determinism is not 'the truth', unless one believes it to be the case, and even then one still has free will and agency whether we realise it or not. By recognising the phenomena of encroaching determinism in any of its forms, and how we might be unwittingly caught or identified in one of its traps, and then dis-identifying from this, we are at least part of the way to securing our release. Paradoxically, as we step back into the witness, observer or I, we become empowered to see what is possible and to take a next step towards something better. As we fully recognise how powerless we are to change a particular set of systems forces, an inner intelligence awakens that knows how to bring about systemic change. For example as I stopped struggling to change the old leadership dynamics within an organisation I was part of, by recognising the particular parental transferences that were being triggered for me by the leaders, I was able to find a very different way of working with these leaders to progress the goals that were important to me.

However, as we know, the awareness that comes from disidentification is not enough. Too much coaching (in common with counselling or therapy) stays too long in awareness building without switching mode towards engaging with or activating the will. As psychosynthesis coaches using trifocal vision, we are always looking for where the *Will* is available, alongside developing awareness or consciousness.

A side note on 'Will'

So far in this book 'the will' has been mentioned frequently in a number of different contexts, and will continue to be so. For those familiar with psychosynthesis, the ways in which we refer to 'the will' should make sense; for others, our use of language may need clarification. In particular, when we refer to *finding* or *activating free will* or *available will* in coaching, what do we mean? By *free* will, we mean the will of the 'higher Self', your true or authentic self; *will* that comes from who we are and is not an unconscious drive or compulsion arising from historical pathologies or from a particular part of your personality (e.g. a subpersonality). Of course, this distinction can be hard to discern, and sometimes we only know free will when we experience it. Acting out of or expressing free will tends to give rise to more free will, so the coach seeks to start with a small step that can give the coachee an experience of their free will in action. When the will is blocked or caught or hijacked by a part of ourselves, even a small step can be challenging. Once the coachee experiences their will through taking a small step, the coach looks to support a slightly bigger step that builds this experience of free will. Thus we speak about finding available will in the way that we might nurture a small flame or candle light into a larger fire, to use an obvious metaphor.

To take our understanding of will further, I now turn to Assagioli's work on this subject, how he viewed this challenge in his day and how well, I believe, his model has stood the test of time, before then building the foundations for working psychologically to develop will with leaders.

The possibility of agency and free will

Assagioli was already well aware of the impact of runaway modern technology on the world in his day and age and of the direction that this might take mankind unless there was a corresponding shift in consciousness (1974, p6):

> Only the development of his inner powers can offset the dangers inherent in man's losing control of the tremendous natural forces at his disposal and becoming the victim of his own achievements. Fundamental among these inner powers, and the one to which priority should be given, is the tremendous, unrealized potency of man's own will.

Assagioli also offered something that few of the neuropsychologists get close to – that alongside the power of the unconscious, our automatic nature, the extent to which we are herd animals and unconsciously part of systems and

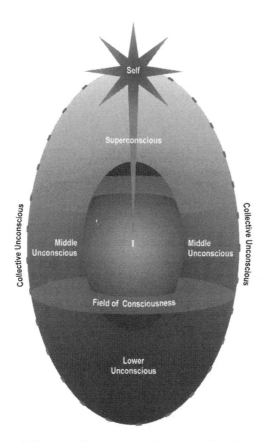

Figure 16.1 Assagioli's egg diagram (Institute of Psychosynthesis version).

societies that influence most of our thinking and behaviour – alongside all this we always have choice and free will. Moreover, Assagioli fully recognises both the collective and individual nature of humanity, because he was able to see those two aspects' deeper and more essential relationship, as represented in his model of the human psyche and Self (see Figure 16.1).

He was therefore able to hold the capacity for individual agency and selfish motivation in right relationship to our need to belong and contribute to the whole.

Assagioli understood that healthy and well-rounded *will* has the capacity to focus and direct the psychological functions of our minds – thinking, feeling, sensation, intuition, imagination, desire, etc. – in service of our higher Self (see Figure 16.2, taken from *The Act of Will*, 1974).

However, much of the time we experience the reverse, with our will blocked or distorted by aspects of our personality and the way that our minds work.

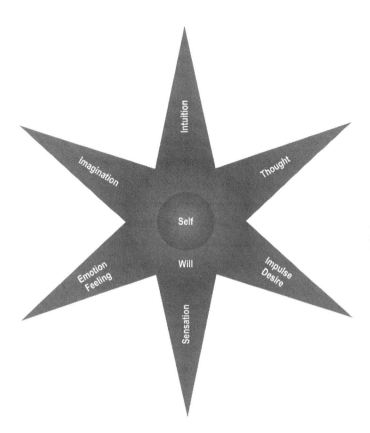

Figure 16.2 Assagioli's star diagram.

We therefore need to work to train our will to direct our psychological functioning.

Assagioli realised that it is not enough to write about will, that our journey to developing the will needs to *'begin by discovering (its) reality and the nature... through its direct existential experience'* (1974, p6). And he offers hope on this journey: *'we are, essentially and genuinely, what we will to be, even if we often fail to manifest it'* (ibid.).

It also seems as if Assagioli lays the ground for coaching in relation to the act of Will (1974):

> The very process of telling our problem to another person helps us to formulate it clearly, to 'objectify' it, so to speak, and thus to understand it better.

> (p159)

There is also the subtle and indefinable but genuine effect of the mere presence of a willing and understanding listener.

(p159)

The most important rule is to formulate, clearly and precisely, the goal to be reached, and then to retain it unswervingly in mind throughout all the stages of the execution, which are often long and complex.

(p179)

It may be said that a 'trifocal vision' is required; that is, the perception and retention in mind of the distant goal and purpose; the survey of the intermediate stages which extend from the point of departure to the arrival; and the awareness of the next step to be taken.

(p184)

Stages of willing – the act of will

The key model in Assagioli's work for engaging the will is his five stages of the act of Will (1974; see Figure 16.3).

This can be described as a simple cyclical model, although in practice it will work differently according to the situation and the scale, often involving cycling back to an earlier stage when progress becomes stuck or blocked. Each of these stages might take days, weeks or months (e.g. creating a new course),

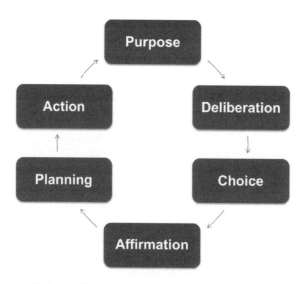

Figure 16.3 Assagioli's stages of the act of will.

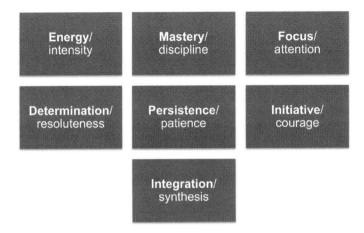

Figure 16.4 Assagioli's qualities of will.

or the whole cycle could be completed in a day (e.g. arranging a social event). We might work with the model explicitly with a coachee or we might use it to reflect upon where the will might be blocked.

In addition to this stage model, Assagioli describes (i) the qualities of the will that might be needed within the activation, expression and realisation of will, as summarised in Figure 16.4; (ii) the key aspects of will – i.e. strong, skilful and good will, as well as transpersonal will; and (iii) his psychological laws in relation to skilful will. Beyond this summary I won't repeat what is well worth reading at source, although I will come back to aspects of will later.

Below I illustrate each of the stages, quoting Assagioli from *The Act of Will*:

Purpose, evaluation, motivation, intention

There are conscious motivations and unconscious motivations; or rather one might say more accurately that there is almost always a combination of the two, in very variable proportions... this is due to the psychological multiplicity that exists in each of us. (1974, Chapter 12, p140)

Deliberation, choice and decision

A decision reached without deliberation, without examining and evaluating all aspects of the question or choice that confronts us, can lead to impulsive, unconsidered, and ill-advised action. (1974, Chapter 13, p151)

Affirmation

*Images constitute another means through which affirmations can be focused;
their dynamic potency is well known. One can use the image, or vision, of what
is wanted as if it were already accomplished.* (1974, Chapter 14, p170)

Planning and programming

*The most important rule is to formulate the goal to be reached clearly and pre-
cisely and then to retain it in mind unswervingly throughout all the stages of the
execution, which are often long and complex.* (1974, Chapter 15, p178)

The direction of the execution

*There is another psychological function which has close connections with those
already mentioned; it is the imagination. Here also there are relationships of
reciprocal action and reaction. Emotions and desires evoke images which correspond to them.*

*The will can encourage — (encourage, not coerce, I repeat)—the intuitive
operation by formulating questions to be addressed to the superconscious sphere,
the seat of the intuition.* (1974, Chapter 16, p189)

I hope this shows how the act of Will constitutes a useful leadership
coaching model in itself. In future writing, I plan to expand upon each of
these stages and show how Assagioli's wisdom is reflected and reimagined in
more recent writing in neuropsychology and neuroscience.

Will and the psychological functions

Assagioli's star diagram (see Chapter 6) shows the will at the centre of and
working through the psychological functions of thinking and feeling, intuition and sensation, imagination and desire. There are two important ways in
which we can take forward our understanding of how this works. The first is
to explore the type or aspect of will associated with each of the psychological
functions more fully. **Strong** will works through *desire*, **skilful** will is a function
of our *thinking* or mental capacity, **good** will stems from our *feeling* nature,
transpersonal will is accessed through our *intuitive* capacity. In the diagram
below, which is adapted from one provided by Alessandra Moretti at our
recent retreat, I have added **creative** will as a function of our *imagination*, and
grounded will associated with our sensation and therefore connection with
earth or nature.

Moretti suggests that each of these psychological functions (along with
their associated aspect of will) can be explored in terms of its own egg diagram
(see Figure 16.5): in other words, we have *pre-personal*, *personal* and *transpersonal* developmental issues, energies and subpersonalities in relationship

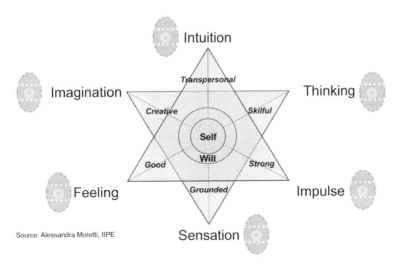

Source: Alessandra Moretti, IIPE

Figure 16.5 Assagioli's psychological functions and aspects of will.

to each of these functions. The skilful coach or therapist can work with a client on their development in each function over time. So for example in my thinking or mental function, I have critical and controlling parts which are located in my pre-personal (echoes of my father); I have analytical and systematic parts within my personal level of consciousness (skills I learned at school for both survival and success); and wise and synthetic parts within my higher unconscious (which require an infusion from my feeling nature to activate). Work I have done in therapy and coaching has been about increasing awareness and choice about which of these parts are in play.

The second way to develop our understanding of how this works is to recognise the dynamic polarities inherent in our psychological functions. This has already been touched upon in the discussion of synthesis and the balance of opposites. The implied polarities are set out in Figure 16.6, with a pyramid as a symbol of the synthesis we are working towards. I have already mentioned the synthesis of something like *compassionate wisdom* that I experienced in relation to healing my split between mind and heart. Another personal example is my imbalance between *intuition* and *sensation* – leading to an overactive capacity for generating visions which are not realistic or grounded. I spent the last 18 years working this one out in relationship to my vision for the château in France that I bought with my wife and we recently sold. One of the gifts of the long struggle in relation to this project was in discovering a level of groundedness through connection to nature and learning to let go of wild plans driven by unresolved parts from my past. I invite you to find some examples for yourself in relation to each of the polarities below. Working with

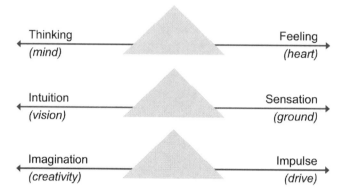

Figure 16.6 Examples of intrapsychic polarity and synthesis.

a client's inner development in such a synthetic way is an advanced skill for a psychosynthesis coach.

At the already mentioned 2019 retreat, Moretti then demonstrated how we can use a variety of techniques to work with each of the psychological functions in relation to will, and specifically for coaching, in relation to achieving a goal or, as she describes it, *magnetising* the goal. Typically, we might use our thinking and feeling capacities to formulate and refine a goal that has come through our intuitive function. The technique summarised in the box below then shows how we might draw upon the other psychological functions to magnetise the goal further.

Magnetising your goal using the psychological functions

- Chose a challenging goal that is important to you
- Imagination – connect with a symbol or image that represents your goal

  - Allow yourself to stay in contact with the energy that emanates from it

- Desire – provides energy for the process and grounds the goal

  - How much and in what way do you desire this? Visualise your desire or connect it with your image

- Sensation – the body becomes informed with energy and joy

  - Where is the desire for this goal located in your body? What is it like to move as if your goal is achieved or coming about?

Bringing will back to centre stage

Finally, I want to briefly reflect upon the overall experience of will in our lives and the lives of our clients, referring back to the discussion about the new determinism and the systemic, societal loss of free will. The questions I want to suggest we need to keep asking are:

- How do we bring Will back to centre stage in our lives and for our clients?
- How do we recognise, nurture and develop free will, for ourselves and our clients?

Often we need to rediscover our 'no' before we can find a true connection with our 'yes'. Assagioli emphasised that often exercising free will is about not doing something as much as about doing something. This is even more the case in our current day and age of sensory overload and continuous stress and pressure from every direction in our lives. Last month I didn't watch any television and wrote this book instead. This month I am looking for a way to lessen my addiction to the smartphone in my pocket. Asking your coachees what they need to say 'no' to before they turn and tune their will towards 'yes' is important.

I will end this chapter with three more questions we can keep asking, and which hopefully this book helps inform:

- Training the will – what techniques can you use?
- Coaching the will – how do we work in the gap to find and activate free will?
- Exercising the will – what does this look like in our lives?

And of course, all of these come within the scope of leadership coaching.

Chapter 17

Psychosynthesis techniques

Which psychosynthesis techniques are most valuable for coaching? How might psychosynthesis coaches draw upon a range of techniques that they can use with their clients?

Two schools

Some readers who are familiar with psychosynthesis might have expected earlier inclusion and more emphasis on techniques in this book than has been the case. This is worth some explanation. I have observed two schools in psychosynthesis practitioners, whether coaches, counsellors or therapists. Practitioners of the first and more traditional school favour the frequent use of techniques as explicit interventions with their clients (in what we earlier called the coachee's space), and indeed Roberto Assagioli seemed to work in this way. Practitioners of the second school favour working more fluidly, flexibly or informally with the client (in what we have called the coaching space), and only occasionally explicitly introduce an intervention.

These two schools might also be described as different styles of working, and I would suggest they can be observed as operating across different modalities, psychologies or approaches within all the helping professions. Here I will state neutrality with respect to these two styles and say that I have observed they both can work for coaches, depending upon your preferences and skills, although in practice I lean towards working primarily in the coaching space and will only occasionally use explicit techniques. Many coaches will find that they move between the different styles according to the specific needs of the situation and their client (as described by the four Cs).

Assagioli was also at pains to explain that the use of any technique must fit the situation and that for the most part *'we use a pragmatic approach and basically strive to respond to the direct needs of the patient (*coachee*), to meet them on the grounds of their more immediate and urgent issues...'* (1965). This topic is expanded upon in a short chapter (2017, p187) by Petra Guggisberg, in which she describes the classification of techniques Roberto Assagioli uses in *Psychosynthesis, a Manual of Principles and Techniques* (1965). In the table

Table 17.1 Techniques in psychosynthesis coaching according to Assagioli categories

Category	Coaching equivalents and examples
1. Inventory phase	Awareness building – *information gathering, including profiling, feedback and journal keeping*
2. Exploring the unconscious: the analytical techniques	Personal development – *getting to know and mastering our personality. Inner exploration of our lower, middle and higher unconscious*
3. Techniques for personal psychosynthesis	Self-actualisation – *working on ourselves to discover our true abilities and higher potentialities*
4. Techniques for transpersonal psychosynthesis	Self-realisation – *recognition and realisation of our true or higher Self*
5. Other techniques *Expressive and anchoring techniques* *Relational techniques* *Further techniques*	Presence, mindfulness, resilience, communication, right-relations, interpersonal – *skills and capacities*

above I have summarised this classification, along with some current coaching equivalents and examples.

Since Assagioli's time, many psychosynthesis practitioners have continued to adapt and develop Assagioli's original techniques as well as to create new ones. There are therefore many good sources of psychosynthesis techniques that can usefully be employed by coaches for working with their clients. Martha Crampton was one of the early pioneers of psychosynthesis life coaching and her writing is rich in the description of useful techniques, including on the use of the imagination and guided imagery and on empowering the will (see Chapter 3 in *The Call of Self*, 2018).

Many years ago, I came across a pamphlet compiled and edited by Thomas Yeomans describing twelve psychosynthesis exercises, which I have found very useful and which can still be found on the *synthesiscenter.org* website. On occasion I have even given this to clients to draw upon for themselves as a way of continuing their personal development beyond our coaching. Other sources of techniques include Piero Ferrucci's work, starting with *What We May Be* (1982), and Kenneth Sorensen's more recent *The Soul of Psychosynthesis* (2016).

Over the last two years PCL has been working in partnership with the IIPE in Italy, running coach training and development programmes for their community of psychosynthesis counsellors in Verona, Turin, Modena and Trento. We have discovered that they place greater emphasis on certain techniques in their work and have enjoyed learning about some of these techniques, which can usefully be employed in coaching. I enjoy the way the Italian psyche seems more attuned to the imagination and intuition, more appreciative of beauty and able to work freely and creatively with imagery and symbols. In addition, as already mentioned in the previous chapter, I like the expanded way they work with the will and the psychological functions and the techniques they are developing to magnetise the goal in coaching using will expressed through the different psychological functions. I had in mind to work together with our Italian colleagues at IIPE to develop their material on psychosynthesis coaching techniques for this chapter, but now feel this is best tackled as a separate project following the publication of this book.

I will now return to the topic of disidentification within psychosynthesis and the use of the disidentification meditation, as well as meditation and visualisation techniques in coaching. The disidentification meditation, variously adapted from an original model by Assagioli (1965), is central to the personal practice of many psychosynthesis coaches, and we use it at the beginning of all our teaching days. Psychosynthesis coaches may also use it in their preparation for every coaching session, to centre themselves and find an inner connection. It can be introduced directly with clients but this should not be done without thoughtful consideration of the coaching context and the coachee. Offer it as an invitation, when you feel a level of trust and understanding has been established in the coaching relationship, and only when your intuition tells you it won't make your coachee uncomfortable. A simple disidentification meditation can be used to take a group or an individual into their inner space, from which a number of other possible pathways open. The inner space can be used to simply reflect more deeply than is normally possible on current issues or recent events, or can be used to engage with the imagination and creativity in an infinite variety of ways, combining too with many other psychosynthesis techniques.

Guided meditations can be directed towards allowing or inviting an image, symbol or word to emerge for the coachee in relation to a theme or topic. They can also be used to enable the coachee to have an inner conversation with or between parts of themselves, sometimes evoking a wise or transpersonal part to offer guidance or insight. There are a number of basic principles about how to direct a guided meditation to make use of archetypal symbols (meadows, mountains, dwellings in woodland clearings, etc.) and these can be read about elsewhere. However, it is important to remember that essentially anyone can guide and support anyone else in simple, flexible and informal ways to enter into an inner receptive space and engage with their imagination in creative and resourceful ways, without drawing upon particular techniques. For the most part less is more (i.e. don't over-elaborate: say as little as is needed and allow space) – what is most important is that the coach or facilitator is attuned to the coachee and sensitive to what is happening in the coaching space.

Mindfulness

This is a good point at which to consider the role and relationship of mindfulness in psychosynthesis coaching. There has been an enormous increase of interest in and practice of mindfulness over recent years in the organisational world and in many ways this can be seen to help open the door to psychosynthesis.

Keith Hackwood (who ran a session on mindfulness as self-care for coaches at our PCL Psychosynthesis Coaching Symposium in 2018) sees psychosynthesis and mindfulness as naturally supporting each other, but also sounds a warning (Hackwood, 2016, np):

> Mindfulness, as we know, is a global phenomenon and precisely because of the scope of its success and far reach, the term itself risks becoming overly diluted or emptied of meaning. Currently Mindfulness is a term applied to clinical and behavioural applications, stress relief, new age workshops, neuroscientific research; it is a core component of the training of managers in some blue-chip companies and all recruits to the US Marine Corps are given Mindfulness training to enhance their resilience. In fact it has been said that Mindfulness today is 'whatever the marketplace decides Mindfulness is', which is an easy thing to say, but masks huge and largely unexplored consequences.

He goes on, having sketched the origins of mindfulness from Buddhist practice, to describe its modern emergence today:

> By and large the practices of Mindfulness as they have entered mainstream globalised and materialist life today, through the secular biophysical and psychological models of Jon Kabat-Zinn and those who followed his work, tend to be 'cool' in nature. That is to say, they cultivate an awareness of mental detachment, of breath body and thought awareness, of disidentification, we might say, seeing 'thoughts as thoughts' not as 'true' or as 'part of my identity'.

This is a secular mindfulness, shedding its spiritual roots and focusing on the measurable benefits of practices adapted for a busy organisational world, and by all accounts successfully delivering important benefits to leaders as a result. There are resonances here both with the disidentification practices touched upon earlier in this chapter and with the somatic path of coaching discussed in Chapter 14. The good news for us is that leaders who might be practising mindfulness techniques will already have had some practice with disidentification. The flipside of this is that some may be tipping over into disassociation, or using mindfulness as an escape from the pressures of work situations without increasing their self-awareness in relation to them.

Mindful coaching is also becoming established as a genre in its own right. Liz Hall (Passmore, 2014) introduces some core mindful practices that coaches might use with clients (e.g. the mindful minute, mindful walking, witnessing our thoughts) as well as her own FEEL model (Focus, Explore, Embrace, Let go) for those seeking to coach mindfully. She also challenges the assumption of goal-orientation in coaching (as with Whitmore's GROW model) and suggests that *'encouraging clients through mindfulness to be more curious, more accepting, less attached to outcome and comfortable with not knowing, can be immensely fruitful, particularly when they are faced with ambiguous and complex worlds to navigate'* (Passmore, 2014, p199).

There is clearly compatibility and synergy between psychosynthesis and mindfulness, and I have witnessed this develop for some of the students on our programmes who come with a mindfulness training background. For most psychosynthesis coaches, mindfulness represents a rich source of methods and techniques which have been organisationally road-tested and which they might incorporate into their coaching practice. At the same time, we would argue that on its own the modern mindfulness approach is not enough – that from the psychosynthesis perspective, mindfulness practice needs a psychospiritual model of the self for teachers or coaches to make sense of experiences emerging from practice, and a coaching model that balances disidentification and self-awareness with activating will.

Chapter 18

Insights from neuropsychology and the implications for psychosynthesis coaches

What should the psychosynthesis coach know about neuroscience? Is neuro-science telling us anything new? How do we reconcile scientific and psycho-spiritual perspectives?

Introduction

Is neuroscience telling us anything new? How do we reconcile scientific and psychospiritual perspectives? Most coaches will have come across neuroscience or neuropsychology in some form or other. Unless you have explored the field extensively for yourself, you may be wondering what there is to learn from this rich new seam of discovery and how you might draw upon it in your coaching practice.

I have approached this topic from the perspective of the psychosynthesis coach, a perspective which values inner inquiry and experiential observation as a valid knowledge path alongside behavioural observation and scientific discovery in the material world. We work with the inner lives of our coaching clients throughout all levels of consciousness and realms of the psyche (e.g. body, feelings, mind, spirit, etc.) as well as their outer lives of action, behaviour and goals. From this perspective, I am asking, is neuroscience:

- telling us what we already know about the mind and human behaviour, by using an explanation of what is going on in the brain?
- telling us something significantly new or different that we should listen to and incorporate in our coaching? or
- telling us that we have got some things wrong and need to work in a new or different way?

The quick answer is: a bit of each of these. To answer this question more fully, I delved primarily into two sources (see Figure 18.1); Paul Brown and Virginia Brown's *Neuropsychology for Coaching* (2012) and Sarah McKay's *Your Brain Health* website, where she unpacks the 'Seven principles of

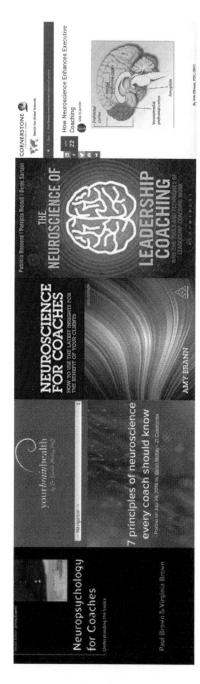

Figure 18.1 Book and blog graphics – neuroscience for coaching.

neuroscience every coach should know' (2018). I also looked at *Neuroscience for Coaches* by Amy Brann (2017), which appears to be doing a similar job to *Neuropsychology for Coaching*, and Deb Elbaum's blog post on 'How neuroscience enhances executive coaching' (2018), which covers similar ground to Sarah McKay's.

I have also drawn from my own reading in the wider field of neuropsychology (e.g. David Eagleman, Thaler and Sunstein, David Rock) and experimental psychology (e.g. Daniel Kahneman, Daniel Goleman, David Brooks) over the last ten years or so (see Figure 18.2). Whatever we may think of neuropsychology, we certainly can't ignore it, and in this chapter I will tell you why.

Overview of neuropsychology for coaching

The neuroscientists and neuropsychologists who are speaking to the coaching profession appear to be doing a combination of three things.

1   Educating us in the neuroscience of how the brain works, for example explaining the mechanics of neurology and brain chemistry and how these determine our functioning and behaviour – *which can be interesting but is not essential for a coach. It depends upon your appetite for the science.*
2   Telling us about neuroscientific discoveries in terms of insights into human nature and how human beings work and the implications of these for coaching – *which is both interesting and important.* Some of this provides scientific evidence to support what we already know from other knowledge perspectives. Some offer new and valuable insights that we should be incorporating in the way we work. This is what I will focus on in this article.
3   Developing a new approach to coaching based directly upon neuroscientific evidence and principles – *so far the attempts to do this that I have seen don't work.* I hope I remain open to new ideas about coaching but will resist those which are blind to underlying philosophical and epistemological biases and inconsistencies. One of the traps of the modern age is how easily science slips into scientism or materialistic reductionism (i.e. only the physical world is real), often without any awareness. To understand this issue more fully I refer back to Wilber's integral model and concept of Flatland as explained in previous chapters. Ignoring or denying one or more of Wilber's four quadrants causes problems (e.g. performative contradictions), particularly when you step outside one discipline (e.g. neuroscience) and attempt to show how this knowledge applies in a broader context (e.g. the coaching profession).

Unfortunately, the extent to which some neuroscientific proponents are aware of the wider knowledge context within which they are contributing their

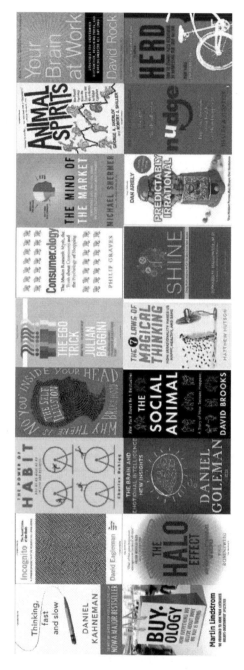

Figure 18.2 Book graphics – neuroscience and neuropsychology.

discoveries is limited. Many are poor at recognising their own assumptions and biases and are therefore prone to making inaccurate or inconsistent assertions (e.g. Wilber's performative contradictions). They are not even very good at recognising other knowledge within their field, or related fields such as experimental psychology.

Many are also poor at distinguishing between (i) the science (does a coach really need to know about how the amygdala works?), (ii) the insights from the science about human nature, our minds, behaviour, relationships, etc. and (iii) the implications of this for leadership and the coaching profession.

Of the sources I read, the best at avoiding these traps and recognising other perspectives was Sarah McKay's blog post (2018), in which she includes some of the science but focuses more on the insights and implications for coaches. Her seven-point summary of Kandel, Cappas and colleagues' thoughts on how neuroscience can be applied to coaching is as follows:

1   Both nature and nurture win.
2   Experience transforms the brain.
3   Memories are imperfect.
4   Emotion underlies memory formation.
5   Relationships are the foundation for change.
6   Imagining and doing are the same (to the brain).
7   We don't always know what our brain is 'thinking'.

These are expanded upon in her post, which is where I recommend you look next to deepen your understanding of this topic. Below I incorporate these and other insights into my own summary.

This is my high-level synthesis of what I take from all the sources mentioned.

Human nature

We need to fundamentally recalibrate our understanding of human nature – for example recognising the primacy of emotions over rationality, and the extent to which we are social animals and relational beings and less individually autonomous than we think.

Brown and Brown (2012) explain how emotions are triggered through chemicals and neural pathways much more quickly than conscious thought, so that our reactions, choices and decisions are largely emotionally driven and post-rationalised.

Experimental psychology shows how systemic cognitive biases make us poor decision makers (e.g. cognitive dissonance, the halo effect, confirmation bias, hindsight-bias, risk aversion, over-optimism), as well as revealing how easily we are influenced by others without realising it (e.g. following fashions, herd behaviour). We are much closer to the animal world and more influenced by our biological and genetic inheritance than we admit.

What is worse is that we are, for the most part, unconsciously blind to our human nature and will continue in a state of self-delusion even when the wider reality has been revealed. This capacity for self-delusion is also pervasive throughout our organisations and societies. Most typically, organisations believe they make rational rather than emotional decisions more than is in fact the case. Societies also tend to assume people make rational decisions based upon the information that's available. Recent global events are shaking us out of this self-delusion. The discoveries of neuropsychology potentially offer an antidote to our tendency for self-delusion, but need to be administered skilfully if they are to work.

Implications for coaching?

Seek to see the individual and the systems that they are part of in relationship, and work to support the coachee to become aware of the human systems they are influenced by.

Hold lightly and be curious about our clients' rationalisations and justifications, helping them to reflect upon their own cognitive biases and emotional undercurrents, and be curious about rationality bias and other collective self-delusions that exist within their organisational system.

Hold a holistic context for your coaching – for example awareness of the whole person including soma, feelings, mind and spirit, all levels of consciousness and unconsciousness, engaging with past, present and future.

There is a wider message about human nature to hold in our awareness, which is well summarised by Michael Shermer (2008): *"Most people misjudge what would make them happy. Happiness stems from love, meaningful work, community participation and spiritual practice. To be happy, engage in these things and support a society that allows others to do the same."*

Anything new to the psychospiritual perspective?

The core models of psychosynthesis, for example Assagioli's models of the psyche and the psychological functions, already provide the theoretical foundations for working with an expanded view of human nature – the new discoveries give us material to work with in shifting consciousness within today's organisational and societal context.

Assagioli (1974, p140) says:

> ...[T]he human tendency to find apparently good justifications for actions that are not good; justifications to ourselves and justifications to others. This tendency could be compared to the pleading of an inner attorney who defends the cause of the more intense urges operating in the unconscious." And also "the knowledge of the existence of these 'lower' elements in ourselves need neither surprise nor depress us; they exist in all human beings!

The mind

Alongside this, at the individual level, our understanding of how the mind works is developing rapidly based upon findings from both brain science and experimental psychology. The headline is that the unconscious, automatic, emotionally-driven and habit-forming part of our mind is much more pervasive and in control than we realise. The conscious, deliberative, slow and energy-consuming part likes to think it is in charge, but for the most part it is not.

Daniel Kahneman describes these two cognitive systems as the fast 'System 1' and slow 'System 2'. Daniel Goleman also recognises two systems that are not always in sync – the low road of immediate emotional response and the high road of rational thought. Sarah McKay (2018, np) summarises the neuroscience as showing that *'unconscious processes exert great influence on our thoughts, feelings, and actions'*, whilst Deb Elbaum (2018, np) emphasises the *'struggle between the amygdala and the prefrontal cortex... also known as the amygdala hijack'* – basically saying that leaders can easily get hijacked by hasty emotional reactions and need to find a way to take a step back and reflect before acting.

Implications for coaching?

Working with an awareness of the 'parts' and supporting the coachee in this awareness is essential for coaching. The most basic distinction between the conscious self on one hand (e.g. System 2) and the unconscious, automatic mind on the other (System 1) is an important starting point. Beyond that, we can look to build the coachee's awareness of a multitude of parts within their consciousness and to see the tensions or conflicts that can arise between them. From a psychospiritual perspective, we are also seeking to develop the capacity to disidentify from these parts (although paradoxically one must recognise and identify them first in order to disidentify) and build our sense of self – the place of awareness from which we can observe our identifications with different parts.

McKay (2018, np) tells us how *'the brain can process non-verbal and unconscious information and information processed unconsciously can still influence therapeutic and other relationships. It's possible to react to unconscious perceptions without consciously understanding the reaction'*. This validates any holistic approaches to coaching in that it endorses that everything going on in the coaching space, whether conscious or unconscious, is relevant and has transformative potential.

Anything new to the psychospiritual perspective?

I'd like to think that we are already working from the principles underlying the truth being discovered in these new ways. However, this new language of the unconscious mind (e.g. Kahneman's Systems 1 and 2) and the evidence base about how it works, can help bring the mainstream with us. Psychosynthesis offers the systemic model of subpersonalities as a way of understanding the nature and relationship of different parts of our personality.

Assagioli (1974, p140) said: *'There are conscious motivations and unconscious motivations; or rather one might say more accurately that there is almost always a combination of the two, in very variable proportions!'* And also: *'We are dominated by everything with which our self becomes identified. We can dominate and control everything from which we disidentify ourselves'.*

Behavioural change

There is both bad news and good news coming out of this field concerning change. On one hand, *'the brain hates change'* (Brown and Brown, 2012, p64) and becomes grooved in habitual responses that require conscious will and repeated practice to regroove.

On the other hand, the concept of *neuroplasticity* (my one concession to the jargon!) explains how the brain is always capable of relearning and developing new behaviours. McKay elaborates the principle (2012, np): *'the areas of our brain associated with emotions and memories… are not hard-wired, they are "plastic". Circuits in our brain change in response to experiences, not just during development…'*

Our brains have a drive towards normalisation, quickly adapting to any new circumstances with new routines that can be consigned to the automatic, unconscious part of brain functioning. In *The Power of Habit* (2013), Charles Duhigg explains how *'habits are actions people first decide to do deliberately and keep doing subconsciously. The "habit loop" has three stages: a "cue" propels a person into a "routine" to reach the goal of a "reward." Understanding how your habits fit these habit loop stages can help you change them'.*

Implications for coaching?

Neuroscience endorses that all relationships, including the coaching or therapeutic relationship, can be important in enabling positive change.

Neuroplasticity confirms that deep change throughout our lives is more readily possible than we thought. For example the long-held assertion that psychological type (e.g. using MBTI) is relatively fixed through our lives has been shown to be inaccurate.

Anything new to the psychospiritual perspective?

Neuropsychology brings something new in terms of understanding how change takes place and what is needed to bring about successful change. This can be combined with the psychosynthesis approach to transforming mindsets (see here) or other more cognitive behavioural approaches such as Kegan's 'immunity to change' (2009).

Amongst other things, psychosynthesis is a psychology of Self and Will. The importance of our will and the role of coaching in developing, finding and activating free will is only increased by the evidence from neuro- and experimental psychology. Without *will*, we are at risk of being lost in a sea of unconscious powerful processes and forces at play at individual, relational and collective levels that are only exacerbated by ever-increasing complexity in modern life. Neuropsychology, as far as I can tell, has nothing useful to say about the will (maybe, like the self, it can't find a place in the brain in which it resides), and in this respect psychosynthesis is still fairly unique as a psychology that helps us to support coachees to find and develop their free will (not just strong, skilful or good will).

Assagioli says about the will: '*the discovery of the will in oneself and even more the realisation that the self and will are intimately connected, may come as a real revelation…*'

Memory and narrative

Our memory is basically faulty! Neuroscience shows how memories, emotions and feelings are closely interconnected neural processes in the brain. Memories are recreated each time we recall them and, as we do so, we weave in new narratives, alongside new emotions and feelings. '*Autobiographical memories that tell the story of our lives are always undergoing revision precisely because our sense of self is too*', as McKay (2018, np) puts it.

Kahneman (2012) tells us how '*people prefer to make simple stories out of complex reality. They seek causes in random events, consider rare occurrences likely and overweigh the import of their experiences*'. He also makes an important distinction between what he calls our two selves – the experiencing self, which lives in the present, and our remembering self, which evaluates the past and decides about our future.

We are also highly selective in our remembering – and yet don't realise it. Bruce Hood (2012), citing Daniel Kahneman, explains that '*we have about 600,000 experiencing moments a month, each of which lasts about 2 or 3 seconds, but most are lost. That is why our memory is always fragmented, and why we often believe so strongly that our recollection is correct when it is not*'.

Implications for coaching?

Gervase Bushe offers some useful perspectives on this topic. In *Clear Leadership* (2010) he speaks to the human inclination to make up stories to fill gaps in our understanding and how we tell these stories to gain agreement for our 'positions'. He shows how common and problematic our partial perceptions and faulty memories can be and how this contributes to interpersonal mush within organisations. Much coaching involves untangling this interpersonal mush for our coachees. Bushe suggests ways in which we can communicate our experience more effectively by more explicitly acknowledging our observations, feelings, thoughts and wants.

The importance of stories or narratives in human life is becoming clearer – they are central to our sense-making and understanding of ourselves. They are therefore key to the coaching process in more than one way. Psychosynthesis has always emphasised the importance of stories, and we use the metaphor of the journey as an important device within our storytelling.

Anything new to the psychospiritual perspective?

I would suggest that the extent of the unreliability and selectivity of our memory is new knowledge. Knowing how our memory and emotions function are closely interconnected in the brain and helps our understanding of how we constantly reshape our memories. Of all the insights from neuroscience, I find those concerning memory to be of greatest potential significance.

As human beings, we are always in the process of developing our own mythology, consciously or unconsciously. By this I mean we are finding meaning and significance in our past and looking for purpose and self-expression in our future. There is an extraordinary and even mystical dimension to this, which we can only touch upon here. We are effectively changing the past in the way we do this, as well as creating the future. That is not to say that we can fictionalise or fantasise the past to our liking, just as fantasising about the future is only useful when we also engage our will. From a psychospiritual perspective, we seek to weave our mythology in ways that are connected with the higher Self, that bring about healing of the past, transformation of the present and inspiration for the future. Importantly, the coach can and should support this process for their clients.

Imagination and creativity

Imagination was one of two psychological functions that Roberto Assagioli explicitly added (the other was impulse or desire) to Jung's four primary psychic functions (sensation, feeling, thought and intuition). The capacity for imagination and creativity has tended to be side-lined by the rational–behavioural bias within our organisations, or at least consigned to specific roles and activities. Neuropsychology is helping to bring it back to centre stage, and it should play a vital role in leadership coaching. Elbaum (2018) speaks about the need for 'whole brain wisdom' by engaging the right hemisphere of the brain (e.g. by drawing upon metaphor and imagery) alongside the analytical left brain, in a process of synthesis with which many leaders are not familiar.

As touched upon with the previous theme of memory, our imagination works in all temporal directions. As Sarah McKay puts it (2018, np): *'consciously or not, we use imagination to reinvent our past, and with it, our present and future'.* She adds *'mental imagery or visualisation not only activates the same brain regions as the actual behaviour but also can speed up the learning of a new skill. Envisioning a different life may as successfully invoke change as the actual experience'.*

Brown and Brown (2012) support this view of coaching as including all temporal domains: *'any client brings to any coaching session… him- or her-Self. The whole of the person is always present in the room. This includes their past, present and future'.*

Implications for coaching?

The value and power of visualisation, imagery and even guided mediation in coaching has been validated by neuropsychology. Psychosynthesis explains the psycho-spiritual principles underlying the efficacy of these tools as well as bringing an expanding repertoire of techniques and ideas for coaching practice.

Anything new to the psychospiritual perspective?

McKay's quote above resonates with Assagioli's words from more than forty years ago: *'images or mental pictures and ideas tend to produce the physical conditions and the external acts that correspond to them'.* Assagioli's psychological laws then take this to a much more sophisticated level: see Chapter 5 in *The Act of Will* (1974). The development and engagement of imagination has always been core to the practice of psychosynthesis and the neuroscientific validation of why it works is very welcome.

Summary

In this chapter I have attempted to synthesise my understanding of key insights from both neuro- and experimental psychology and suggest some implications for coaching. In doing so, I have sought to minimise the scientific jargon and use the language of the mind rather than the brain. At the same time, I have shown how these discoveries can combine with and enhance a psychospiritual approach to coaching. I have illustrated, with quotes from Roberto Assagioli's work (he described himself as a scientist of the spirit), the extent to which there isn't necessarily much new wisdom here for those working from a psychospiritual perspective. At the same time, it does add something important by helping build a richer and more detailed picture of what is going on and providing valuable material which the coach can use in today's organisational and leadership contexts.

Neuro- and experimental psychology offer fascinating insights and new awareness about human nature, our minds and behaviour. But it cannot give us a coaching methodology in its own right, because as coaches we are working with people, not brains. My argument is that in order to work with the implications of these new sciences, which primarily concern what is going on within the human being (our minds, being, consciousness, etc), you need a methodology and indeed a core psychology, such as psychosynthesis, that works with the inner subjective dimension. To seek to build a purely neuroscientific methodology for coaching seems strangely irrelevant and unnecessary – a bit like trying to design a robot that can paint art, when human beings can already do this better than a robot is ever likely to. There is a need for perspective about how neuroscience can be useful and for the objective sciences to find their proper place alongside the subjective disciplines rather than seek to take over the whole territory.

This leads into a wider argument: that any holistic approach to coaching leaders and seeking to bring about beneficial change in organisations and society needs to be *integral*, in the sense that it recognises all four of Wilber's essential perspectives: objective and subjective, inter-subjective and inter-objective. So, for example by combining the neuropsychological *objective* perspective, the psychospiritual *subjective* perspective, the developmental *inter-subjective* perspective and the systemic *inter-objective* perspective we can develop a powerful new approach, not just for dealing with the complexities of leadership coaching but for tackling the really serious emergent societal leadership issues of today. I will develop this theme in my future writing.

Chapter 19

A new synthesis and the future of psychosynthesis coaching

Has this book achieved a new synthesis within the umbrella of psychosynthesis coaching? What might a new synthesis look like? How can the community of psychosynthesis coaches grow and prosper?

Coach as alchemist

What does it feel like to consider yourself as an alchemist when working as a coach? How does this shift your attitude, perspective or mindset towards coaching? What space might this open up for you in relationship to the coachee? Maybe you will find less need for conscious control and more trust of the unconscious process. The alchemist needs to be able to hold paradox, to work with the interplay of opposites and hold seeming contradictions. I turn to the description of the alchemist from Rooke and Torbert's stages of leadership development (2005), which includes *'the interplay of awareness, thought, action and effect. Transforming self and others'*, and *'anchoring in inclusive present, seeing the light and dark in situations; works with order and chaos'*. This seems an apt description of how the psychosynthesis coach might be seeking to work.

At the same time, I remind myself of the need to stay grounded and avoid the traps of grandiosity or inflation. One of the reasons I like the alchemy metaphor is that, despite the aura of mystery, the original purpose was to create gold from base metal, something very practical and material. Our challenge as coaches is to stay open to mystery (or that which is beyond the control of our conscious minds). We need to stay grounded in the practical and pragmatic and help our clients do the same whilst continuously holding the creative tension for ourselves and our clients. To quote Roberto Assagioli *'What is synthesis? It could be defined as a dynamic, creative balance of tensions'*.

Where now?

How is psychosynthesis coaching developing for the future? Most broadly, we are working towards creating a vision and version of psychosynthesis that is more fit for purpose in the leadership and organisational world.

It is worth considering whether we can and should describe psychosynthesis as *evolutionary,* in terms of Laloux's paradigms. My answer for now is that psychosynthesis coaches and other practitioners need to develop their capacity to work from an *evolutionary* paradigm. Mostly this doesn't look like anything in particular, because the *evolutionary* perspective is always looking at the health of the whole system, and when working in the system *evolutionary* practitioners tend to blend in or adapt according to what works in the environments and situations in which they find themselves. I mentioned earlier that Laloux's work has spawned a number of *evolutionary* (or *teal*, to use his associated colour) networks and movements. The danger with these is that *evolutionary*/teal is becoming a place to get to rather than to come from, another paradigm that is better than the others, rather than a place or perspective that dis-identifies from and transcends the limitations of our worldviews.

So how do we reposition psychosynthesis? By the very act of bringing psychosynthesis more fully to leadership coaching and working with leaders in organisations (e.g. with the Institute's MA in organisational and leadership coaching, our PGCPLC, 5DL coaching and coaching supervision courses), I believe we are already beginning to evolve an organisational-friendly and *evolutionary* version of psychosynthesis. I have a couple of thoughts on what will help with this:

1   We need to continue developing versions and expressions of psychosynthesis that are more accessible and attractive to the organisational and leadership world. This will involve continuing to unpick some of the therapeutic and *pluralistic* biases which have become too identified with psychosynthesis. A good way to do this is to return to Roberto Assagioli's source material and rebuild towards the future (as also advocated by Kenneth Sorensen) by drawing upon the perspectives I have highlighted – i.e. systemic, development and somatic, as I have attempted to do in this book.

2   At the same time, we need to allow a plurality of versions of psychosynthesis to become more clearly delineated and develop alongside each other. There has been enough falling out between factions within the psychosynthesis community over the years, so we should now work towards bridge building within the wider international community, through the acceptance and encouragement of diversity and exchange. Associations such as the EFPP in Europe and the Association for the Advancement of Psychosynthesis (AAP) can play an important role in this.

Ending... and beginning the future

This book presents a multi-perspectival exposition of psychosynthesis coaching. What I hope I have set out is a dynamic, emergent and developing model of psychosynthesis coaching. It is work in progress, and a continuing personal and professional journey for myself and others. Central to this approach is the work of Roger Evans and the core model of trifocal vision, which is about how to coach the *being* – learning to hold a psycho-spiritual context beyond the mind, to use your heart as the resonator of Self. This is a seemingly simple idea, but difficult to practise.

Leadership coaching as an emerging profession is far from simple, encountering many layers of challenges and complexities. In this book, I have explored the many dimensions and aspects of leadership coaching, with the intention of describing an extended model of psychosynthesis coaching which has evolved through our PCL coaching programmes and continues to be informed and supported by involvement with the wider psychosynthesis community.

Ultimately coaching is about practice, and reflecting upon and learning from that practice. Ironically coaching is most often a one-to-one activity and might be viewed as a lonely profession; however, there are many ways in which the coach can engage and benefit from relationships with other professionals. Supervision is obviously important (and group supervision has particular advantages); so is continuing personal and professional development, along with exchange and support through communities of practice.

My continuing motivation is to see more and more psychosynthesis coaches supporting leaders during this critical period of human evolution. I believe that key to this will be to create a strong, vibrant and active community of practice for psychosynthesis coaching. I hope this book will contribute to that coming about.

We keep moving. I end with three quotes: one by Assagioli, one by Graves and starting with one from a blog post about evolution:

> We are moving! Carter Phipps quotes the biologist-theologian Pierre Teilhard de Chardin as saying, and in more ways than one. But in what direction? Is there a trajectory to evolution? In conversations with a variety of people across disciplines, Phipps discerns a general direction (without a firm destination) of increasing complexity, creativity, and convergence, with a heightening capacity to reflect upon these trends, as they manifest both internally and externally.
>
> (Curtis Ogden (2012, np))

> The psychology of the adult human being is an unfolding, ever-emergent process marked by subordination of older behavior systems to newer, higher order systems. The mature person tends to change his psychology continuously as the conditions of his existence change… Man's nature is emergent. What man is, cannot be seen before. We can see it only insofar as it has been revealed to us by his movement through the levels of human existence.
>
> (Clare Graves (1970, p133))

Life is movement, and the superconscious realms are in continuous renewal. In this adventure we move from revelation to revelation, from joy to joy. I hope you do not reach any stable state. A stable state is death.
Roberto Assagioli

(quoted by Ferrucci, 1982, p126)

Sense, *love* and respond.

Afterword

Sitting at my desk at home in the Drôme Provençale, preparing the final manuscript of this book to send to the publisher, I notice the need to add a few more words. Over the last month or so the world as we have known it has been turned upside down by the coronavirus pandemic and here in France we are five weeks into 'lockdown'. For me personally (whilst always being aware of those less fortunate or at risk), this forced recess or retreat has been something of a blessing, not just granting time to catch up with all sorts of projects, including completing this book, but also the opportunity to pause and reflect, to immerse in my surroundings and to seek connection with the spirit of peace. New projects emerge, not least learning how to run our courses and support leaders and coaches online. I have also started a new series of blog posts, which are giving new shape and direction to my next book, on evolutionary leadership, already signposted a few times in these pages. I don't want to repeat any of that here but I do want to add a few thoughts about change, coaching and leadership.

Often commented on is how the rate of change has sped up these last few weeks – for example how quickly governments have taken steps they would never have previously considered, how we have individually changed many behaviours previously taken for granted, and how much of our world has rapidly learned to work from home using Zoom. Coaches, in particular, are adapting to remote meeting, if they hadn't already, and from a straw poll of my colleagues there are no intrinsic barriers to working at the greater depth described in this book using online methods.

What life and society will all look like when we have fully emerged from this crisis is unknown and uncertain, but alongside danger there is opportunity to reshape and recreate our world. Within this re-emerging world, I believe there is a growing need for a psychospiritual psychology that supports working at the depths needed to heal the past as well as with the heights of purpose, meaning and values. At our psychosynthesis coaching symposium in February 2020, Petra Guggisberg Nocelli presented a session (see the PCL website, www.psychosynthesiscoaching.co.uk/videos/) called *'Psychosynthesis – a psychology whose time has come'*, and I see this title as even more true in our new emergent world.

The call for the kind of coaching this book is about will be greater than ever and the capacity for leadership at all levels to *sense, love and respond* will need nurturing. I hear a particular call to bring psychosynthesis coaching into the domain of political, societal and community leadership.

Looking back at the book I have written, rather than forwards from the preface and introduction I wrote most of two years ago, I notice a few things that I want to mention:

The way in which different parts of the book have come together from other material has created a variability in style, for which I apologise to the reader.

Some of the feedback I received on the draft suggested I cut back on the number of models and theories. I'm afraid I have not done this, mostly to satisfy my obsession for completeness and partly to get some of them out of my system. This is particularly the case with the three chapters on *Personal and Professional*, which together form the comprehensive guide on personal development that I couldn't find elsewhere and which I believe is needed by coaches. I hope that readers who found any chapter heavy going skipped to the next one to find a topic of more interest.

A word about the case stories that I added late on to illustrate practice and bring the material to life. These are drawn from my own experiences in leadership coaching, but are more mythically truthful than based upon factual accuracy. My wife Diana commented that many of the stories seem quite similar, to which I agreed and added that we tend to draw clients towards us that fit a pattern or support our own needs to grow. Your stories of psychospiritual coaching may be quite different.

Finally, the bibliography that follows contains more than the references relating to the text of the book. I have included books on psychosynthesis, coaching and leadership that have influenced me and contributed to my learning about this wider topic. I hope the longer list is helpful. I have also added some web links which I hope are a useful resource. To find these as links, as well as other resources which I will continue to add to, please visit our website below.

Aubyn Edward Howard
La Touche, April 2020
www.psychosynthesiscoaching.co.uk

References and bibliography

Aquilina, Eunice (2016), *Embodying Authenticity – A Somatic Path to Transforming Self, Team and Organisation,* London: Live It Publishing.

Assagioli, Roberto (1965), *Psychosynthesis*, London: Thorsons.

Assagioli, Roberto (1974), *The Act of Will*, London: Aquarian Press.

Assagioli, Roberto (1991), *Transpersonal Development*, London: Aquarian Press.

Assagioli, Roberto (circa 1974), *The Superconscious and the Self*, Source: unknown, Handout by The Psychosynthesis Trust, London.

Assagioli, Roberto (2018a), *Unity and Diversity*, Source: Assagioli Archives: Florence, Translated by Gordon Symons.

Assagioli, Roberto (2018b), *Balance and Synthesis of Opposites*, Source: Assagioli Archives: Florence, Translated by Gordon Symons.

Assagioli, Roberto (2018c), *May the Spirit of Peace Spread Everywhere*, Source: Assagioli Archives: Florence, Translated by Gordon Symons.

Bachkirova, Tatiana (2011), *Developmental Coaching: Working with the Self,* Maidenhead: Open University Press.

Bader, Michael (2009), *The Difference Between Coaching and Therapy is Greatly Overstated,* in *Psychology Today*, April 15, 2009.

Barratt, Richard (2014), *Evolutionary Coaching*, Lulu Publishing Services.

Beck, Don and Cowan, Chris (1996), *Spiral Dynamics*, Oxford: Blackwell.

Belbin, R. Meredith (2004), *Management Teams* (2nd edition), Oxford: Elsevier.

Bertalanffy, Ludwig von (1969), *General Systems Theory*, New York: George Braziller.

Bijlani, Ramesh (2014), *Psychology – Study of the Soul, Mind or Behaviour*. Blog post: www.speakingtree.in/blog/psychology-study-of-the-soul-mind-or-behaviour.

Bluckert, Peter (2006), *Psychological Dimensions of Executive Coaching,* Maidenhead: Open University Press.

Bly, Robert (1988), *A Little Book on the Human Shadow,* New York: HarperCollins.

Boud, David, Cohen, Ruth and Walker, David (1993), *Using Experience for Learning*, Buckingham: Open University Press.

Brann, Amy (2017), *Neuroscience for Coaches,* London: Kogan Page.

Bridges, William (1995), *Managing Transitions,* London: Nicholas Brealey.

Brooks, David (2011) *The Social Animal*, London: Short Books.

Brown, Paul and Brown, Virginia (2012), *Neuropsychology for Coaching,* Maidenhead: Open University Press.

Buckingham, Marcus and Clifton, Donald (2005), *Now Discover Your Strengths (StrengthsFinder),* London: Simon and Shuster.

Bueno, Julia (2010), *Coaching: One of the Fastest Growing Industries in the World Today*, in Psychology Today.

Bushe, Gervase (2010), *Clear Leadership,* Mountain View, CA: Davies-Black.

Cook-Greuter, Susanne (2004), *Making the Case for a Developmental Perspective,* online paper: www.cook-greuter.com/Making%20the%20case%20for%20a%20 devel.%20persp.pdf.

Critchley, Bill (1998), The *Role* of the *Management* Consultant in the *Change Management Process,* in *Management Consultancy: A Handbook of Best Practice,* edited by Philip Sadler, London: Kogan Page.

Curtis, Adam (2016), *HyperNormalisation* (Film, BBC).

Diamond, Jared (1997), *Guns, Germs and Steel: The Fates of Human Societies,* New York: W.W. Norton.

Downey, Myles (2014), *Effective Modern Coaching: The Principles and Art of Successful Business Coaching,* London: LID Publishing.

Duhigg, Charles (2013), *The Power of Habit,* London: Random House.

Earls, Mark (2009), *Herd,* Chichester: Wiley.

Einzig, Hetty (2017), *The Future of Coaching,* Abingdon: Routledge.

Elbaum, Deb (2018), *How Neuroscience Enhances Executive Coaching,* blog post: www. cornerstone-group.com/2018/04/22/how-neuroscience-enhances-executive-coaching/.

Eriksson, Eric (1982), *The Life Cycle Completed,* London: WW Norton.

Evans, Roger (2020), *Five Dimensions of Leadership,* Hendon: Creative Leadership Publishing.

Evans, Roger and Russell, Peter, (1989), *The Creative Manager,* London: Unwin Paperbacks.

Evans, Joan (Ed) (2009), *Core Principles in Psychosynthesis Psychology Applied to Coaching, Module I,* London: Institute of Psychosynthesis.

Ferrucci, Piero (1982), *What We May Be: The Vision and Techniques of Psychosynthesis,* New York: Jeremy P. Tarcher/Penguin.

Firman, Dorothy (Ed) (2018), *The Call of Self,* Amherst: Synthesis Center Press.

Firman, John and Gila, Ann (2002), *Psychosynthesis,* New York: SUNY.

Fisher, Dalmar, Rooke, David and Torbert, William (2000), *Personal and Organisational Transformations.* London: McGraw-Hill.

Fowler, James (1995), *Stages of Faith,* New York: HarperCollins.

Gardner, Howard (1983), *Frames of Mind: The Theory of Multiple Intelligences,* New York: Basic Books.

Goldsmith, Neal (2010), *Psychology – The Study of the Soul?,* blog post: www. psychologytoday.com/us/blog/psychedelic-healing/201011/psychology-the-study-the-soul.

Goleman, Daniel (1996), *Emotional Intelligence,* London: Bloomsbury.

Goleman, Daniel (2007), *Social Intelligence,* London: Bloomsbury.

Graves, Clare (1970), *Levels of Existence, An Open System Theory of Values, Journal of Humanistic Psychology,* Fall 1970, Vol. 10 No.2, pp. 131–155.

Gray, David, Garvey, Bob and Lane, David (2016), *A Critical Introduction to Coaching and Mentoring,* London: Sage.

Greenleaf, Robert (1977), *Servant Leadership,* Mahwah: Paulist Press.

Greiner, Larry (1988), *The Five Phases of Growth,* Harvard Business Review, May-Jun 1998.

Hackwood, Keith (2016), The Moisture of Compassion – Psychosynthesis, Mindfulness & the Luminosity of Mind – online paper: www.keithhackwood.com.

Hall, Liz (2013), *Mindful Coaching: How Mindfulness Can Transform Coaching Practice*, London: Kogan Page.

Hämäläinen, Raimo and Saarinen, Esa (Eds) (2007), *Systems Intelligence in Leadership and Everyday Life*. Espoo: Systems Analysis Laboratory, Helsinki University of Technology.

Handy, Charles (2015), *The Second Curve,* London: Random House Books.

Hardy, Jean (1996), *A Psychology with a Soul,* Totnes: Woodgrange Press.

Harford, Tim (2012), *Adapt: Why Success Always Starts with Failure,* London: Abacus.

Harris, Thomas A. (1969), I'm OK, You're OK, New York: Harper and Row.

Harrison, Roger (1995), *Consultant's Journey: A Dance of Work and Spirit*, London: McGraw-Hill.

Harryman, William (2009), *Robert Kegan & Lisa Lahey - Immunity to Change (Review & Overview)*, blog post: http://integral-options.blogspot.com/2009/12/robert-kegan-lisa-lahey-immunity-to.html.

Hawkins, Peter and Shohet, Robin (2012), *Supervision in the Helping Professions*, 4th edition, Maidenhead: Open University Press.

Hawkins, Peter and Turner, Eve (2020), *Systemic Coaching: Delivering Value Beyond the Individual*, Abingdon: Routledge.

Heider, John (1985), *The Tao of Leadership*, Aldershot: Wildwood House.

Hellinger, Bert (1999), *Acknowledging What Is*, Phoenix: Zeig, Tucker.

Heron, John (1990), *Helping the Client,* London: Sage.

Heron, John (1992) *Feeling and Personhood: Psychology in Another Key,* London: Sage Publications.

Hodge, Alison et al. (2015), Supervision for Executive Coaching: Supervisor as Journey Companion, paper for APECS Symposium 2015 (unpublished pdf).

Hood, Bruce (2012), *The Self-Illusion: Why There is No You Inside Your Head,* London: Constable.

Horowitz, Mark (2014), *The Dance of We – The Mindful of Love and Power in Human Systems,* Amherst, Massachusetts: Synthesis Center Press.

Howard, Aubyn (2015) Bringing a *P*sycho-spiritual *P*erspective to *E*xecutive *C*oaching, paper for APECS Symposium 2015 (unpublished pdf).

Howard, Aubyn (2016), *The Influence of Leadership Paradigms and Styles on Innovation*, Chapter 19 in *Value Creation in the Pharmaceutical Industry*, edited by Alexander Schuhmacher, Markus Hinder and Oliver Gassman, Reutlingen: Wiley.

Howard, Aubyn (2017a), *The Leadership Gap,* LinkedIn post: www.linkedin.com/pulse/leadership-gap-aubyn-howard/.

Howard, Aubyn (2017b), *Therapy and Coaching – Challenging the Orthodoxy*. LinkedIn post: www.linkedin.com/pulse/coaching-therapy-challenging-orthodoxy-aubyn-howard/.

Howard, Aubyn (2017c), *The Somatic Path of Coaching*, blog post: www.psychosynthesiscoaching.co.uk/somatic-path-coaching-working-body-mind/.

Howard, Aubyn (2018), *An Evolving Model of Psychosynthesis Coaching,* Unpublished paper for the Institute of Psychosynthesis.

Howard, Aubyn and Elliott, Paul (2017), *Trifocal Vision*, p 6–8 in PGCPLC Unit One Course Study Guide (unpublished pdf).

Huston, Jean (2013), *The Leadership Dilemma*, blog post: http://jeanhoustonfoundation. org/social-artistry/the-leadership-dilemma/.

International Coach Federation (ICF) website (2018), *Core Competencies*, https:// coachfederation.org/core-competencies.

Jaworski, Joseph (1996), *Synchronicity: The Inner Path of Leadership*, San Francisco: Berrett-Koehler Publishers.

Kahneman, Daniel (2012), *Thinking, Fast and Slow*, London: Penguin.

Kegan, Robert and Lahey, Lisa (2009), *Immunity to Change*, Boston: Harvard Business School Publishing.

Kets de Vries, Manfred (2006), *The Leader on the Couch*, Chichester: Wiley.

Kets de Vries, Manfred (2016), Self-Secure Leaders and the Role of Attachment, (http://knowledge.insead.edu).

Kline, Nancy (1999), *Time to Think*, London: Ward Lock.

Kotter, John (1999), *Leading Change*, Boston: Harvard Business School Publishing.

Kubler-Ross, Elizabeth (1969), *On Death and Dying,* New York: Simon and Schuster.

Laloux, Frederic (2014), *Reinventing Organisations*, Brussels: Nelson Parker.

Lee, Graham (2003), *Leadership Coaching*, London: CIPD.

Lencioni, Patrick (2002), *The Five Dysfunctions of a Team*, San Francisco: Jossey-Bass.

Loevinger, Jane (Ed) (1998) *Technical Foundations for Measuring Ego Development*, Mahwah: Lawrence Erlbaum Associates.

Luft, Joseph (1963), *Group Processes – An Introduction to Group Dynamics*, Palo Alto: National Press.

Luft, Joseph (1969), *Of Human Interaction: The Johari Model*, Palo Alto: National Press.

Machon, Andrew (2010), *The Coaching Secret*, Harlow: Pearson Education.

Martin, Roger (2007), *The Opposable Mind,* Boston: Harvard Business School Publishing.

Maslow, Abraham H. (1968), *Towards a Psychology of Being*, New York: Van Nostrand Company.

Maslow, Abraham H. (1971), *The Farther Reaches of Human Nature*, New York: Penguin.

Maslow, Abraham H. (1943), *A Theory of Human Motivation,* originally published in the 1943 *Psychological Review*, number 50, page 838.

Maslow, Abraham H. *(*1970), *Motivation and Personality* (2nd edition), New York: Harper & Row.

McKay, Sarah (2018), *Your Brain Health, Seven Principles of Neuroscience Every Coach Should Know*, blog post: https://drsarahmckay.com/7-principles-neuroscience-every-coach-know/.

Millichamp, Stacey (2018), Transpersonal Dynamics, Forres: TransPersonal Press.

Mishra, Pankaj (2016), *Welcome to the Age of Anger*, The Guardian, 8 December.

Nocelli, Petra Guggisberg (2017) *The Way of Psychosynthesis: A Complete Guide to the Origins, Concepts, and the Fundamental Experiences, with a Biography of Roberto Assagioli*, Maryland: Synthesis Insights.

Nevis, Edwin C. (1991), *A Gestalt Approach to Organisational Consulting*, New York: Gardener Press.

O'Neill, Mary Beth (2007), *Executive Coaching with Backbone and Heart* (2nd edition), San Francisco: Jossey-Bass.

Ogden, Curtis (2012), *Leadership in a New Age*, blog post at: http://interactioninstitute. org/author/curtis/.

Oshrey, Barry (2007), *Seeing Systems*, San Francisco: Berrett-Koehler.

Palmer, Helen (2012), *Psychosynthesis in the South Pacific*, Institute of Psychosynthesis monograph no 10.

Palmer, Stephen and Whybrow, Alison (Eds) (2008), *Handbook of Coaching Psychology,* Hove: Routledge.

Passmore, Jonathan (Ed) (2014), *Mastery in Coaching: A Complete Psychological Toolkit for Advanced Coaching,* London: Kogan Page.

Passmore, Jonathan (Ed) (2015), *Excellence in Coaching: The Industry Guide* (3rd edition), London: Kogan Page.

Passmore, Jonathan, Brown, Hazel and Csigas, Zoltan (2017), *The State of Play in European Coaching & Mentoring, Executive Report 2017.*

Peltier, Bruce (2010), *The Psychology of Executive Coaching*, New York: Routledge.

Phipps, Carter (2012), *Evolutionaries*, New York: HarperCollins.

Piaget, Jean (1954), *The Construction of Reality in the Child*. New York: Basic Books.

Plotkin, Bill (2008), *Nature and the Human Soul*, Novato: New World Library.

Ramsay, Jay (2017), *Alchemy: The Art of Transformation*, Dorset: Archive Publishing.

Rock, David (2009), *Your Brain at Work,* New York: HarperCollins.

Rodenburg, Patsy (2008), *The Second Circle*, London: WW Norton.

Rooke, David and Torbert, William (2005), S*even Transformations of Leadership*, Harvard Business Review, April 2005.

Rosenzweig, Philip (2010), *The Halo Effect,* New York: Free Press.

Senge, Peter (1990), *The Fifth Discipline,* London: Century Business.

Senge, Peter, Scharmer, C. Otto, Jaworski, Joseph and Flowers, Betty Sue (2005), *Presence: Exploring Profound Change in People, Organizations and Society*, London: Nicholas Brealey.

Shaw, Patricia (1997), *Intervening in the shadow systems of organizations: consulting with a complexity perspective*, Journal of Organizational Change Management, Vol 10 No 3.

Shermer, Michael (2008), *The Mind of the Market*, New York: Henry Hold.

Silvester, Keith and Wignall, Helen (2018), Adaptive Leadership in a VUCA World, unpublished paper for the 2018 Psychosynthesis Coaching Symposium.

Simpson, Steve, Evans, Joan and Evans, Roger (2013), *Essays on the Theory and Practice of a Psychospiritual Psychology, Volume 1*, London: Institute of Psychosynthesis.

Simpson, Steve, Evans, Joan and Evans, Roger (2014), *Essays on the Theory and Practice of a Psychospiritual Psychology, Volume 2,* London: Institute of Psychosynthesis

Smith, Eliot, Mackie, Diane and Claypool, Heather (2007), *Social Psychology* (3rd edition), Hove: Psychology Press.

Smith, Robb (2016), *The Morning After*, blog post: https://integrallife.com/morning-after/.

Smith, Simon (2000), *Inner Leadership,* London: Nicholas Brealey.

Sorensen, Kenneth (2009), *Integral Psychosynthesis: Integral Perspectives on Psychosynthesis*, Masters thesis: https://kennethsorensen.dk/en/integral-psychosynthesis-a-comparison-of-wilber-and-assagioli/.

Sorensen, Kenneth (2016), *The Soul of Psychosynthesis*, s.l.: Kentaur Forlag.

South Africa College of Applied Psychology (2014), author unknown: *What's the Difference Between Counselling and Coaching?* blog post: www.sacap.edu.za/blog/management-leadership/whats-difference-counselling-coaching/.

Stacey, Ralph (1996) *Complexity and Creativity in Organisations*, San Francisco: Berrett-Koehler.

Starkey, Ken and Hall, Carol (2012), *The Spirit of Leadership*, chapter in *The Spirit of Leadership: New Directions in Leadership Education*, edited by Ken Starkey and Carol Hall, Boston: HBR Press.

Stewart, Iain and Joines, Vann (1987), *TA Today*, Nottingham: Lifespace.

Strozzi-Heckler, Richard (2014), *The Art of Somatic Coaching*, Berkeley: North Atlantic Books.

Thaler, Richard H. and Sunstein, Cass, (2009), *Nudge*, London: Penguin.

Todorovic, Natasha and Cowan, Chris (2005), Graves and Maslow: Levels of Existence and Hierarchy of Needs Compared, blog post: https://humergence.typepad.com/the_never_ending_quest/2006/03/graves_and_masl.html.

Torbert, Bill (2014), *Vertical vs. Horizontal Leadership Development*, blog post: www.williamrtorbert.com/vertical-vs-horizontal-leadership-development/.

Turner, Eve and Palmer, Stephen (Eds) (2018), *The Heart of Coaching Supervision*, Abingdon: Routledge.

Van der Kolk, Bessel (2015), *The Body Keeps the Score*, London: Penguin.

Vaughan Smith, Julia (2015), *What has Trauma Got To Do with Coaching? Or Coaching To Do with Trauma?* APECS symposium paper.

Vaughan Smith, Julia (2019), *Coaching and Trauma*, London: Open University Press.

Wade, Jenny (1996), *Changes of Mind*, New York: SUNY Press.

Wheatley, Margaret (1992), *Leadership and the New Science*, San Francisco: Berrett-Koehler.

Whitmore, Diana (2000), *Psychosynthesis Counselling in Action*, London: Sage.

Whitmore, John (1992), *Coaching for Performance: Growing People, Performance and Purpose* (1st edition), London: Nicholas Brealey.

Whitmore, John (2009, *Coaching for Performance: Growing People, Performance and Purpose* (4th edition), London: Nicholas Brealey.

Whitmore, John (2017), *Coaching for Performance: Growing People, Performance and Purpose* (5th edition), London: Nicholas Brealey.

Whittaker Dunlop, Connie (2017), *The Success and Failure of the Coaching Industry*, 5th October, Forbes.com.

Whittington, John (2016), *Systemic Coaching & Constellations* (2nd edition), London: Kogan Page.

Whyte, David (2009), *The Three Marriages – Reimagining Work, Self and Relationship*, New York: Riverhead Books.

Wilber, Ken (1999), *Integral Psychology*, in The Collected Works of Ken Wilber, Volume Four, Boston: Shambhala.

Wilber, Ken (1999), *One Taste, The Journals of Ken Wilber*, Boston: Shambhala.

Wilber, Ken (2009), *Integral Spirituality*, Boston: Integral Books.

Wilber, Ken (1983), *Eye to Eye*, Boston: Shambhala.

Wilber, Ken (2000), *A Theory of Everything*, Dublin: Gateway.

Young Brown, Molly (2004), *Unfolding Self: The Practice of Psychosynthesis*, New York: Helios Press.

Zohar, Danah and Marshall, Ian (2000), *SQ – Spiritual Intelligence, the Ultimate Intelligence*. London: Bloomsbury.

Online resources and links

See and hear

Roberto Assagioli: www.youtube.com/watch?v=e9rVWAxE2hQ
Piero Ferrucci: www.youtube.com/watch?v=Vhp2–nMZCw
John Whitmore: www.youtube.com/watch?v=BRLKHjGlwm4
John Whitmore: www.youtube.com/watch?v=7-D6CnaQUuw
Peter Hawkins: www.youtube.com/watch?v=lJ9AEftb8YY
Gervase Bushe: www.youtube.com/watch?v=0BzttEvFUmE
Frederic Laloux: www.youtube.com/watch?v=GxGGkrtKZaA
Frederic Laloux: www.youtube.com/watch?v=gcS04BI2sbk
Daniel Kahneman: www.youtube.com/watch?v=XgRlrBl-7Yg
Ken Wilber: www.youtube.com/watch?v=NQ_HsQkBkJA
Roger Evans and Petra Nocelli: www.youtube.com/watch?v=I1GDE6fnY0s
Petra Guggisberg Nocelli: www.youtube.com/watch?v=Aw3_ETUF5R8

Useful organisations

Psychosynthesis Coaching Limited: www.psychosynthesiscoaching.co.uk
Institute of Psychosynthesis: www.psychosynthesis.org
Psychosynthesis Trust: www.psychosynthesistrust.org.uk
Istituto di Psicosintesi: www.psicosintesi.it
Istituto Internazionale Psicosintesi Educativa: www.counselingpsicosintetico.org
EFPP: psychosynthesis.net/about-efpp/
APECS: https://apecs.org
ICF: www.coachfederation.org.uk
AC: www.associationforcoaching.com/pages/home
EMCC: www.emccouncil.org
Coaching at Work: www.coaching-at-work.com
GoodReads: www.goodreads.com
GetAbstract: www.getabstract.com
Harthill (The Leadership Development Framework): http://www.harthill.co.uk

About the author

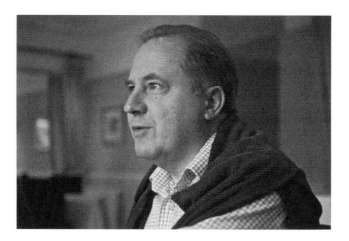

Aubyn Howard is the co-founder (with Paul Elliott) of Psychosynthesis Coaching Limited. Aubyn holds an MA in Psychosynthesis Psychology with the London Institute of Psychosynthesis and an MSc in Change Agent Skills and Strategies with the HPRG at Surrey University. He draws upon more than 30 years' experience as an organisational consultant, facilitator, educator and coach, supporting transformational change and leadership development within all sizes of organisation, across many different sectors and national cultures. Certified Spiral Dynamics and NLP practitioner, APECS Accredited Executive Coach and a Psychosynthesis Coaching Supervisor. Aubyn lives in France with his wife Diana.

Career and experience

After a brief career in the teaching profession, he worked in the Merchants Group for 17 years, becoming Strategy Director before going independent in 1999. Aubyn's focus is on facilitating development within individuals, teams and

*organisations, bringing together psychological, cultural, behavioural and sys-
temic perspectives. Aubyn continues some organisational client work alongside
developing other leadership coaches through PCL's educational courses.*

Academic CV

- Module author and tutor for MSc in management consultancy at Surrey
  University (1999–2001)
- Supervisor and tutor for the MA in psychosynthesis organisational and
  leadership coaching (2011–2015)
- Programme director of the postgraduate certificate in psychosynthesis
  leadership coaching (2015–present)
- 'The Influence of Leadership Paradigms and Styles on Pharmaceutical
  Innovation', Chapter 19 in Schuhmacher, A. and Betz, U.A.K. (2016)
  Value Creation in the Pharmaceutical Industry, Wiley
- *Author of two chapters in* The Call of Self *(2018): Chapter 4: Therapy
  and Coaching – Challenging the Orthodoxy. Chapter 15: The Alchemy of
  Coaching.*
- Papers for 2015 and 2017 APECS Symposiums. Regular blog on PCL
  website and LinkedIn.

Index

Printed in Great Britain
by Amazon

60253125R00140